Law in Optometric Practice

Applie...

Steve Taylor

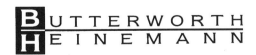

BUTTERWORTH
HEINEMANN

OXFORD   AUCKLAND   BOSTON   JOHANNESBURG   M.

D1077088

Butterworth-Heinemann
Linacre House, Jordan Hill, Oxford OX2 8DP
225 Wildwood Avenue, Woburn, MA 01801-2041
A division of Reed Educational and Professional Publishing Ltd

ℛ A member of the Reed Elsevier plc group

First published 2002

British Library Cataloguing in Publication Data
A catalogue record for this book is available from the British Library

ISBN 0 7506 4578 4

For information on all Butterworth-Heinemann
publications visit our website at www.bh.com

100789
344.0419

Produced and typeset by Gray Publishing, Tunbridge Wells, Kent
Printed and bound by Martins the Printers, Berwick on Tweed

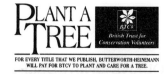

Contents

Acknowledgements

I would like to thank all those who have helped by providing information to support this text, the professional organisations: the Association of Optometrists, College of Optometrists, Federation of Ophthalmic and Dispensing Opticians and the General Optical Council. In particular, Helen Stanforth, Helen Bowman and Bob Hughes have supplied information often at short notice! I would like to thank Caroline Makepeace and Robert Edwards at Butterworth-Heinemann for their patience and understanding. Finally I would like to thank Lorraine for all her support during the production of this text.

Law in Optometric Practice – Introduction

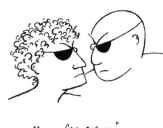

"An eye for an eye ..."

The eyes and the law have been intimately connected since the time of Hamurabi. Probably the most quoted and best-known legal phrase is a translation of Hamurabi's code of ethics 'an eye for an eye and a tooth for a tooth'. As Hamurabi is taken as the father of the legal system, then the eyes were, even in his days, considered important enough to be included at the birth.

The importance of the eye in society has maintained its high status. The early practitioners of ocular health ran a very great risk of loss of limb and financial ruin. In the Greek codes of law a practitioner would lose his hands if he were to treat a nobleman and cause the loss of an eye. Should the eye belong to a servant, then the practitioner was expected to replace the servant if the treatment resulted in the loss of an eye. In view of the state of understanding (or lack of it) of surgery and intra-ocular disorders, and the inability to see into the eye before commencing treatment, it is surprising that anyone ventured into the risky business of ophthalmology. The advent of modern techniques and changes in the legal system have obviously helped to produce a healthier number of optical specialists, all with both hands intact!

The optical profession in Europe, as separate from the professions of medicine and ophthalmology, can obviously be traced back to the invention of spectacles. It is difficult to put a date on this as the initial years of spectacle production are shrouded in mystery. Marco Polo, reporting on his travels in China in 1275, mentioned that people wore glasses before their eyes for reading. The first evidence of the development of spectacles in Europe dates their invention to about AD 1280. Documents still exist in Venice, however, which refer to the manufacture of a form of spectacles which appeared in the first half of the thirteenth century. This evidence contradicts the general theory that a Florentinian, Salvino Degli Armati, was the inventor. He was credited with the invention in an inscription said to exist in a tomb in the church of Santa Maria Maggiore:

> Here lies Salvino Degli Armati son of Armato of Florence inventor of eyeglasses. May God forgive his sins. AD 1317.

The tomb is no longer in existence, and recent research has cast doubt upon the validity of the inscription.

It would seem that spectacles were definitely in use by 1282, when a reference in the records of the Abbey of Saint Bavon le Grand indicates that a priest called Nicholas Bullett used spectacles when signing an agreement. It may be, however, that spectacles were reinvented by a Dominican monk who kept the invention a secret for commercial reasons. The evidence to support this comes from a reference in the Lenten Sermon on 23 February 1305 in the church of Santa Maria Novella in Florence. The sermon was given by Giordarno de Rivalto, who credited Friar Della Spina with the invention.

As a legal body, spectacle makers in Europe were first introduced into a Guild by Louis XI of France in 1465. At this time the Guild also included haberdashers and upholsterers. This was changed in 1581 when Henry III granted a new guild consisting of mirror makers, toy makers and spectacle makers. The first German Guild of spectacle makers was established in Nuremberg in 1577. The Guild had the function of maintaining law and order within its profession.

In Britain the spectacle makers were incorporated by a Royal Charter granted by Charles I on 16 May 1629. The Charter, giving permission to form the Spectacle Makers Company, provided the opportunity to create laws and to produce a profession. It became a 'closed shop', with the Company granting only certain people, who had trained for their craft, permission to practise their trade. The original Charter gave the Court of the Spectacle Makers the power to make 'laws and statutes, decrees, ordinances and constitutions for the good rule and government of the Fellowship and craft'.

The Spectacle Makers Company began to lose a little control in the late eighteenth century, and the British Optical Association (BOA) was eventually formed as an organized body in 1895. The function of the BOA was to improve standards within the profession, and an examination system was quickly established. Not to be outdone, the Spectacle Makers introduced their own examinations in 1898. The Spectacle Makers Company examinations at this time were mainly practical and biased towards the manufacturers of lenses and frame materials. Sight testing was not incorporated into the examination syllabus until 1904.

Since these early days of the formation of the nucleus of a profession there has been a rapid rise in the standards of education and a requirement for registration. More recently the professional bodies have been rationalized to form a single examining body for optometry – the College of Optometrists. Further development and co-operation between professionals has been called for by the General Optical Council following the Optical Services Audit Committee report. On the consumer side, greater awareness of the services available and a better understanding of legal rights have led to a more demanding patient.

To meet these changes various legislative orders have been introduced. The advances in the law relating to ocular health directly relevant to the practising optometrist will be outlined in the chapters that follow bringing the reader up to the current situation.

A Brief Introduction to the British Legal System

As far as the optometrist is concerned there are two main sources of legal circumstance that can potentially affect them in their professional role. The first is action under common law and the second action under legislation. While the consequences and procedures for the two types may be very similar the development of the two legal situations has been very different. As an introduction a brief history of the development of the two forms of law are outlined below.

Common Law

This can trace its roots back to the Middle Ages when the Normans through their system of feudal land tenure introduced a central government and laws common to all parts of England and later Wales. Under the system all land belonged absolutely to the Crown and persons holding land did so merely as tenants of the Crown. The Crown therefore had absolute powers over how the land and its occupants were treated. Consistency in legal matters was maintained by itinerant Royal judges who, in the King's name, travelled to all parts of the country settling disputes which related mainly to the possession of land. Gradually these judges were called upon to extend their jurisdiction to criminal matters and were able to lay the foundation of a Common Law of property and crime.

By the thirteenth century a number of changes to the system had steadied the development of Common Law. These changes mainly were instigated through the Barons who were protecting their self interests by attempting to reduce the powers of the Royal Court in favour of their own profitable feudal courts that had been set up. Restrictions imposed by the Barons meant that Common Law continued to develop but along very conservative lines. One of the developments was for Common Law to expand from just criminal and property matters to include Law of Contract and Law of Tort. These two additions were to deal with civil wrongs that did not amount to a criminal offence.

By the Middle Ages four main types of court had evolved:

1 Communal Courts applying local customary law. These declined as Common Law developed.
2 Seignorial Courts operated by the feudal landlords for their tenants. These also declined as Common Law developed.
3 Ecclesiastical Courts dealing with discipline of the clergy and matrimonial and testamentary matters. These courts declined after the Reformation and matrimonial and testamentary jurisdiction moved to the High Court in the nineteenth century.

4 Royal Courts which included courts of Common Law and Equity. Within this umbrella a number of specialist areas were developed:
   (a) the Courts of Assize dealing with criminal matters
   (b) the Court of the King's Bench dealing with both criminal and civil actions involving the Crown
   (c) the Court of Common Pleas dealing with civil action between subjects particularly relating to land
   (d) the Court of Exchequer dealing with revenue matters
   (e) the Court of Exchequer Chamber dealing with appeals from other Common Law Courts.

In the nineteenth century Parliament made extensive reforms to the judicial system and administration of the law that ended many of the anachronisms in Common Law. By combining the administration of Common Law with that of Equity the Judicature Acts from 1873 to 1875 removed a final source of inconsistency and conflict.

Common Law is still the basis of modern English law and continues to develop by the Doctrine of Precedent by which judges apply established or customary rules of law to new cases as they arise. It is said to be 'unwritten law' because there is no comprehensive set of statutes, judgments, etc. that may be applied in a particular case.

Legislation

Legislation is formed by regulations laid down by a body constituted for the purpose, such as the British Parliament. Enacted laws of this type are called statutes. Legislation may be direct (e.g. Acts of Parliament) or indirect or delegated such as Statutory Instruments (SIs) laid down by a Minister of the government under power given by Act of Parliament. Currently British Parliament is normally the supreme legislative body in the UK although in certain areas ultimate decisions may rest with the European Parliament. Delegated legislation is considered to be as binding as Parliamentary legislation. There is a clause however where if it is considered that if anyone with delegated authority has exceeded their powers the laws laid down can be considered as void. This is the doctrine of *ultra vires* and has on occasions formed the basis of discussion within optometry.

Parliament consists of three essential components:

* the Sovereign
* the House of Lords
* the House of Commons.

Proposals for legislation must be placed before both Houses in the form of Bills. If approved by both Houses a Bill is then placed before the Sovereign for Royal Assent at which point the Bill becomes an Act of Parliament.

There is a difference between the legal systems in England, Wales, Scotland and Northern Ireland all of which have their own Courts and their own National Assemblies able to make their own legislation covering certain aspects.

The need for delegated or subordinate legislation has increased as the time constraints on Parliament have been tightened and greater and greater technical knowledge is required in some areas to provide the fullest debate. The General Optical Council (GOC) can therefore provide specialist expertise to delegated legislation proposed by the Minister for Health and is called upon from time to time to make comments on or even to draft SIs.

There are a number of legal systems with which the practitioner may come into contact besides criminal and civil actions. The Privy Council, which at one time wielded most of the governmental powers, is now largely formal and advisory in function. It is composed mainly of cabinet ministers, former ministers and Law Lords and led by a member of the Cabinet. It is a source of delegated legislation in the form of Orders in Council that may affect practice.

Administrative Tribunals associated with the health service are part of the complaints' procedure. If a complaint concerning a practitioner failing to comply with NHS Terms of Service were to be considered serious enough and could not be resolved informally then it would be referred to an Administrative Tribunal. The powers of such a Tribunal are restricted and ultimate decision, on appeal, lies with the Secretary of State.

The GOC would fall within the classification of a Domestic Tribunal whose function is to maintain discipline among members of a profession and to protect the public. Its role was established by the Opticians Act 1958 (revised and updated 1989) and it has delegated powers to make regulations in certain specified areas. The Privy Council does have power of veto in certain areas and did use these powers during debate on changes to the contact lens regulations in 1984/85. The GOC however acts to maintain standards of practice in accordance with the duties laid down in the Opticians Act 1989. It has the power to remove a practitioner's name from the register effectively preventing them from sight testing.

The College of Optometrists has no statutory function but is effectively an organization of members of the profession that offers guidance on good practice for the public benefit. The examination functions of the College of Optometrists are carried out on behalf of the GOC who regularly satisfy themselves that adequate standards are being met. As with any organization there are agreed rules and failure to comply may result in an individual's membership of the organization being withdrawn. Unlike the consequences of removal from the GOC register, leaving the College will not prevent a practitioner from testing sight.

The National Health Service

Introduction

Since the acceptance by parliament of the ideals of a health service for all within the community, optometry has had a role. Initially that role was seen as one of 'supplementary' to the Hospital Eye Service (HES). Gradually, however, as it became clear that the HES was never going to reach a point where it would be able to satisfy the demand for eye care, the optometrists became part of the General Ophthalmic Services (GOS). Essentially individual optometrists, through Health Authorities (HAs), enter into a contract with the National Health Service (NHS) to provide eye care, to those eligible, for a negotiated fee paid by the state. At the outset, this service was provided without charge to the patient, but in recent times this has changed and eligibility to health service facilities for eye examinations and appliance supply through optometric practices has been restricted.

It is the development of the NHS that has played such a major role in the changes within optometry. Some would say that the link with the NHS has stifled the development of a fundable examination only service for eyes and has placed optometry in the situation in which it finds itself today, largely unappreciated for the eye care provided. While this may be true, it is also the development of the NHS that allowed practitioners to become well established in the early days, and to concentrate on the patient examination without the commercial pressures of today's environment and to stimulate the demand for eye testing. Whatever the truth of the matter, optometry and the NHS are less interwoven now than at any time since the 1946 Act, and it is interesting to review how the 'marriage' between the two has slowly broken down.

Establishment of the NHS

On 6 November 1946, an act to establish a comprehensive health service for England and Wales was passed by parliament. This was the birth of the NHS. According to the National Health Service Act 1946, it was the:

> ... duty of the Minister of Health ... to promote the establishment in England and Wales of a comprehensive health service designed to secure improvement in the physical and mental health of the people of England and Wales and the prevention, diagnosis and treatment of illness, and for that purpose to provide or secure the effective provision of services in accordance with the following provisions of the Act.

The National Health Service Act 1946 was set up according to four principles:

1 The health service should be financed by taxes and contributions paid when people were well rather than by charges levied on them when they were sick; and the financial burden of sickness should be spread over the whole community.

2 The health service should be truly national, aiming at providing the same high quality of service in every part of the country.
3 The service should provide full clinical freedom to the doctors working within it.
4 The health service should be centred upon the family doctor team providing the essential continuity to the health care of each individual and family, and mobilizing the services needed.

Since the National Health Service Act 1946, the following further relevant legislation has been enacted:

- National Health Service (Scotland) Act 1947
- Health Services Act (Northern Ireland) 1948
- National Health Service (Amendment) Act 1949
- National Health Service Act 1951
- National Health Service Act 1952
- National Health Service Act 1961
- Health Services and Public Health Act 1968
- National Health Service Reorganisation Act 1973
- National Health Service Act 1977
- Health Services Act 1980
- Health and Social Security Act 1984
- Health and Medicines Act 1988
- Opticians Act 1989
- National Health Service and Community Care Act 1990
- Health Authorities Act 1995
- National Health Service (Primary Care) Act 1997
- Health Act 1999.

The gradual changes brought about by these acts have produced a present-day situation that bears only a slight resemblance to that originally proposed. The changes can be best demonstrated by a rapid resume of the principal acts.

National Health Service Act 1946

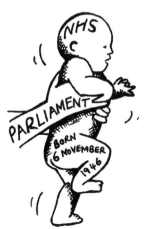

Under the original 1946 enactment the administration of the health service was divided into four main branches:

1 The minister, as central planner and co-ordinator, would oversee each of the other branches and plan to integrate these as a whole, and would also accept ultimate responsibility for the services.
2 The hospital and specialist services were to be administered on a regional basis by hospital boards, the exception being the teaching hospitals. To ensure maximum efficiency, the hospitals were further divided into local groups managed by hospital management committees.
3 Domiciliary care (not treatment) was to be provided by the local authorities and included:
  (a) the care of expectant mothers and young children
  (b) domiciliary midwifery

(c) home nursing and health visiting
(d) vaccination and immunization
(e) ambulance services and health centres
(f) the care of physically and mentally handicapped.

4 The general practitioner (GP) services were to be administered by the executive councils established under Part IV of the National Health Service Act 1946, Section 31. Normally the executive councils were to be responsible for the services in the area of a local HA, ensuring that there were sufficient practitioners within their area and administering the remuneration and terms and conditions of service.

In order to assist the minister and to give advice on general matters relating to the administration of the health services the Central Health Services Council was established. In a further effort to maximize efficiency the minister had the right to constitute standing advisory committees to provide specialist information on any specific aspects of the health services as and when it was required. These advisory committees fell into nine groups:

1 Standing Medical Advisory Committee
2 Standing Dental Advisory Committee
3 Standing Pharmaceutical Advisory Committee
4 Standing Ophthalmic Advisory Committee
5 Standing Nursing Advisory Committee
6 Standing Maternity and Midwifery Advisory Committee
7 Standing Mental Health Advisory Committee
8 Standing Tuberculosis Advisory Committee
9 Standing Council and Radiotherapy Advisory Committee.

This, then, provided a sound central administration with the ability to examine carefully any specialist problems that might arise.

In the case of the executive councils, a specialist knowledge was even more readily available. The 25 members of an executive council included: seven members appointed by the local medical committee, three members appointed by the local dental committee and two members appointed by the local pharmaceutical committee.

The local representative committees were formed where the minister was satisfied that for the areas of any executive council, the committees were representative of

- the medical practitioners of the area
- the dental practitioners of the area
- the people providing pharmaceutical services in the area.

Representatives of the optometrists and dispensing opticians providing supplementary ophthalmic services in the area were not formally recognized until the 1949 Act. In spite of the recognition shown by the act, ophthalmic membership of an executive council was not forthcoming until the Health Services and Public Health Act of 1968.

Role of the Minister of Health

Under the terms of the National Health Service Act 1946, the minister was given the ultimate responsibility for the health service and was seen as the co-ordinator. The responsibilities and the position of the minister could be summarized as follows:

1 Central controller and planner, basing decisions on the information from the central council and the standing advisory committees.
2 Maker of detailed rules, regulations and orders (subject to the control of parliament) by which the health service was to be controlled.
3 Securer of parliamentary sanction for continued financing of the service, with added responsibilities of monitoring costs of the service, approving expenditure and reporting back to Parliament on matters of expenditure.
4 Default and enquiry powers which gave sanction to decisions and requests.
5 To acquire and own, on behalf of the government, land needed for the purposes of the act.
6 Responsible for all new legislation relating to the health services and many other matters relating to welfare and environmental health.

This vast degree of responsibility made the minister the integral part of the NHS, without whom the various units could not function to provide a comprehensive and truly National Health Service.

The National Health Service Act 1946 Relating to Optical Services

The ophthalmic services to be offered under this legislation were to be known as the supplementary ophthalmic services. The reason for this title was that the original ideal of the health service providing full eye care within the confines of the HES could not be achieved, and the Minister of Health established the Eye Services Committee whose function was to look at and report on:

1 The status, the scope of work and the designation of opticians in the final form of the national ophthalmic services as envisaged in the original National Health Service Act 1946.
2 The criteria to be applied when selecting opticians for appointment in the (temporary) supplementary eye services.

The committee was composed of representatives of ophthalmologists, medical practitioners and ophthalmic and dispensing opticians. The role of opticians in the proposed NHS was established on the basis of the Eye Services Committee report published in May 1947. As a result of the report, the Central Professional Committee for Opticians was established in November 1947, to consider all applications to work in the supplementary ophthalmic services. Any optician applying to work in the health services was required to give evidence of qualification and of adequate experience.

By the time the health service was operational in July of 1948, it became a duty of the newly formed executive councils to establish services in connection with the diagnosis and treatment of disease or defect of the eyes and the supply of optical appliances. To ensure an adequate specialist service the duties of the executive council in the field of ophthalmics were to be exercised on behalf of the council by a committee called the ophthalmic services committee.

Regulations were made to include provision for:

1 The preparation and publication of lists of medical practitioners, of ophthalmic opticians and of dispensing opticians who undertook to provide supplementary ophthalmic services.
2 Conferring the right of inclusion in the appropriate list on all having an eligible qualification.
3 Conferring on any person the right to choose who should test his or her eyes and who should supply the prescribed appliance.
4 The removal from the list of ophthalmic or dispensing opticians undertaking to provide supplementary ophthalmic services the name of any ophthalmic or dispensing optician who had never provided or who had ceased to provide such services.

The National Health Service Act 1946 also resulted in the establishment of an optical Whitley Committee, the purpose of which was to negotiate salaries for hospital opticians, fees for opticians working part time within the HES and fees for opticians working in the supplementary ophthalmic services.

Essentially, the original legislation set out to make provisions such that everyone was eligible for free eye examination and free spectacles within the supplementary ophthalmic services. Before this a relatively small percentage of people had been eligible for certain optical benefits by way of the additional benefit provisions of the National Health Insurance Acts.

Health Services and Public Health Act 1968

The Health Services and Public Health Act 1968 was intended:

> to amend the National Health Service Act 1946 and the National Health Services (Scotland) Act 1947, and make other amendments connected with the National Health Service; to make amendments connected with local authorities' services under the National Assistance Act 1948; to amend the law relating to notifiable diseases and food poisoning; to amend the Nurseries and Child Minders Regulation Act 1948; to amend the law relating to food and drugs; to enable assistance to be given to certain voluntary organisations; to enable the Minister of Health and the Secretary of State to purchase goods for supply to certain authorities; to make other amendments in the law relating to the public health; and for purposes connected with the matters aforesaid.*

As can be seen, this was a wide-ranging piece of legislation.

---

*Minister of Health. Ministers are chosen by the Prime Minister and appointed by the Crown on the Prime Minister's advice. The Minister of Health is in charge of the Department of Health, and is responsible for all decisions taken by the department.

Secretary of State for Health and Social Security. This is one of the Crown's Principal Secretaries of State, responsible for the administration of the Health and Social Security Department, constitutionally, they act as a channel of communication between the Crown and its subjects.

Effect of the Health Services and Public Health Act 1968 on Optical Services

The effect of this legislation on the supplementary ophthalmic services was beneficial. The executive councils had their membership increased from 25 to 30, and for the first time one ophthalmic optician and one dispensing optician acted as representatives nominated from the local optical committee (LOC).

This legislation also put the ophthalmic services on a permanent footing; it became known as the GOS and not the supplementary ophthalmic service. The old ophthalmic services committee, whose job (on behalf of the executive councils) had been to assess the qualifications of those wishing to offer ophthalmic services in areas where they were needed, could thus be dissolved. (This was included under the terms of the new Health Services and Public Health Act.) In addition, Section 18(3) provided an amendment to the National Health Service Act 1946, allowing for the provisions of GOS at health centres by ophthalmic medical practitioners, ophthalmic opticians and dispensing opticians.

Finally, ophthalmic and dispensing opticians were defined as follows:

1 'Ophthalmic optician' means a person listed in either of the registers, maintained under Section 2 of the Opticians Act 1958, of ophthalmic opticians, or bodies corporate enrolled in the list, maintained under Section 4 of the Opticians Act 1958, of such bodies carrying on business as ophthalmic opticians.
2 'Dispensing optician' means a person listed in the register, maintained under Section 2 of the Opticians Act 1958, of dispensing opticians, or bodies corporate enrolled in the list, maintained under Section 4 of the 1958 Opticians Act, of such bodies carrying on businesses as dispensing opticians.

National Health Service Reorganisation Act 1973

It was decided that, despite the amendments of the 1968 Act, and the fact that the NHS had certainly lived up to the four principles upon which it is based, there was a certain need for streamlining. Four objectives had to be met in the reorganization:

1 The uniting of existing separate services, followed by their integration at local level.
2 The establishment of close links between the unified service and the public health and social services provided by local authorities.
3 The maximum responsibility for administering the service consistent with national plans and priorities should be placed on area HAs. There should be strong local and professional participation and community involvement in the running of the services in any particular district.
4 The provision for effective central control over money spent on the service and to obtain maximum value.

It was decided that the NHS should be provided and financed by central government. This meant that a boundary had to be drawn between the types of services administered by the HA and those administered by the local authority.

The National Health Service Reorganisation Act was eventually placed on the statute books in 1973. The new Act still placed the minister at the head of the services but required also that the following should be provided:

1 Hospital accommodation.
2 Other accommodation for the purposes of any service provided under the National Health Service Acts.
3 Medical, dental, nursing and ambulance services.
4 Such other facilities for the care of expectant and nursing mothers and young children as are considered appropriate as part of the health service.
5 Such facilities for the prevention of illness and for the care of persons suffering from illness as are considered appropriate as part of the health service. (These facilities replaced the arrangements made by the local HAs under Section 12 of the Health Services and Public Health Act 1968.)
6 Such other services as are required for the diagnosis and treatment of illness.

In addition to the above provisions, there should be arrangements for regular and adequate checks of schoolchildren for both medical and dental health. Also a regular family planning service was established.

The local administration set-up was now directly under the control of the minister and in the form of:

1 Regional HAs.
2 Area HAs.
3 Area HAs (teaching) if any tuition was undertaken at the hospitals within the area.

In this administrative system the minister could direct any of the authorities to carry out any function on his behalf related to the National Health Services Acts. The regional HA could direct an area HA within its own region to carry out any function relating to the National Health Service Acts, with the proviso that the minister could counter such directive.

It became the task of the area HAs to establish family practitioner committees (FPCs) to replace the executive councils and administer the provision of general:

1 medical services
2 dental services
3 pharmaceutical services
4 ophthalmic services.

The FPC comprised:

1 Eleven members appointed by the area HA.
2 Four members appointed by the local authority (or jointly if two or more local authorities were entitled to appoint members).

3 Eight members appointed by the local medical committee of whom one must be an ophthalmic medical practitioner.
4 Three members appointed by the local dental committee.
5 Two members appointed by the local pharmaceutical committee.
6 One ophthalmic optician appointed by the LOC.
7 One dispensing optician appointed by the LOC.

In addition to these, formal recognition was given to a committee where the Secretary of State was satisfied that it was formed for the regional HA, as representative of any of the following:

1 Medical practitioners of the region.
2 Dental practitioners of the region.
3 Nurses and midwives of the region.
4 Registered pharmacists of the region.
5 Registered ophthalmic and dispensing opticians of the region.
6 Any group of representatives of other categories providing services.

Effect of the National Health Service Reorganisation Act 1973 on Optometrists

As far as the ophthalmic services were concerned, this legislation had little effect. The LOC became a firmly established part of the area HA and gave the optical profession a voice in the administrative system at local level. The only other change was simply one of name, with the executive council becoming the FPC without any alteration in the optical representation or duties.

National Health Service Act 1977

This act was issued in order:

> to consolidate certain provisions relating to the health service for England and Wales; and to repeal certain enactments relating to the health service which have ceased to have any effect.

Part I of the Act dealt with services and administration at national and local levels. It set out the duties of the Secretary of State as regards health services. Also under Part I the Secretary of State was required to establish councils termed community health councils, and it was a statutory duty that all parts of area HAs be included within the district of a community health council. The composition of these councils was outlined in Schedule 7 of the Act, and the duties were:

1 To represent in the health service, the interests of the public in their district.
2 To perform other functions as laid down within the schedule. These other functions were to include:
    (a) to visit and inspect premises controlled by the relevant area HA
    (b) to consider matters relating to the operation of the health service within their district and advise the area HAs

(c) to prepare and publish reports on the operation of the health service within their district.

Part II of the National Health Service Act 1977 dealt specifically with general medical, general dental, general ophthalmic and pharmaceutical services. As far as the GOS were concerned, the act required that every area HA arrange for medical practitioners with the prescribed qualifications and ophthalmic opticians to provide a service for the testing of sight and for suitably qualified ophthalmic and dispensing opticians to supply optical appliances.

Section 39 required that lists be drawn up of suitably qualified practitioners who would undertake to provide GOS. Any person suitably qualified wishing to be included in the appropriate list should be so included. It also made provision for the general public to choose whomsoever they wished to test their eyes and whomsoever they wished to supply their appliance. A final note related to removal of the name of anyone included in the list who had never provided or who had ceased to provide such GOS in the area.

Part III of the Act discussed other powers of the Secretary of State relating to the health service. Regulations relating to the changes for dental or optical appliances were laid down in Section 78, that referred to para. 2 of Schedule 12 to this Act. The schedule gave details of the interpretation of the term 'current specified cost' as related to spectacle frames. It also listed details of exemptions from normal costs including children under 16 years of age or receiving full-time education in school. The information was related to the terms of service for ophthalmic opticians as laid down in Statutory Instrument (SI) 1974/287.

Part IV related to property and to finance for the HAs.

Part V detailed the terms of service of a Health Service Commissioner (HSC) for England and an HSC for Wales.

Part VI related to miscellaneous items not falling within these other categories.

Health Service Act 1980

The effect of this legislation was to replace the area HAs with local district HAs.

Health and Social Security Act 1984

This Act introduced the framework for a new set of terms of service that form the basis of those currently in use. It also withdrew the range of NHS frames and lenses that were available to eligible individuals and introduced in their place a voucher system for the provision of appliances.

Organizationally the status and constitution of the FPCs were amended.

For optics this act was a major change to the way services had previously been supplied and should be considered as fundamental to the development of optical services.

Health and Medicines Act 1988

Another fundamental change to GOS was introduced by this Act that withdrew the right of all individuals to an NHS sight test. The Act restricted eligibility categories for those entitled to an NHS sight test and moved the service towards privatization.

Opticians Act 1989

This was a consolidation Act to pull together the legislation that had been enacted since the original act of 1958. This Act will be discussed in more detail in Chapter 7.

National Health Service and Community Care Act 1990

Following circulation of a discussion document from the NHS 'Working for Patients' FPCs were replaced by Family Health Service Authorities (FHSAs) upon implementation of the National Health Service and Community Care Act 1990. It was the responsibility of the FHSA to continue to administer the services previously provided by the FPC and also to extend responsibility in relation to:

1 planning
2 development and monitoring of primary health care services
3 collaboration with other service agencies and local authority Social Services Departments
4 implementation of the NHS white paper 'Caring for people' and the National Health Service and Community Care Act 1990.

The Act also changes the membership of the FHSA which in future will consist of:

1 chairman appointed by the Secretary of State
2 Four professional non-executive directors (one from each of the following service professions):
  (a) GP
  (b) dentist
  (c) pharmacist
  (d) nursing
3 five generalist non-executive directors appointed by the Regional HA
4 General Manager of FHSA as an Executive Director.

Health Authorities Act 1995

This Act of Parliament abolished Regional HAs, District HAs and FHSAs and replaced them with HAs and Special HAs. As far as optometry is concerned the effect of this was purely to change the title of the authority controlling local arrangements.

National Health Service (Primary Care) Act 1997

An amendment was made to the Opticians Act 1989 via this 1997 Act. The effect of the amendment was minor but provided slightly more flexibility for referral although this has now been further updated with the introduction of SI 1999/3267 (see Chapter 5 for further details).

Also the National Health Service and Community Care Act 1990 was amended through this Act to specify that provision of ophthalmic services by a person on the ophthalmic list fell within the context of a service under NHS contract.

Health Act 1999

Between December 1997 and October 1998 the government published a series of papers on its proposals for the NHS in England, Scotland and Wales. The documents were:

- Cm3807 The new NHS.
- Cm3811 Designed to Care.
- Cm3841 Putting Patients First.
- HSC 1998/113 A First Class Service.
- Partnership in Action (a discussion document).
- Quality Care and Clinical Excellence (a consultation document).
- Partnership in Improvement.

Following on from these the Health Act 1999 received Royal assent in June 1999. It had far reaching consequences for the NHS and some specific amendments to regulations affecting optometry. The main purpose of the act was to make changes to the way in which the NHS is run. GP fund-holding was abolished and the act paved the way for the establishment of new statutory bodies (Primary Care Trusts).

A new body was formed aimed at improving quality of care. The Commission for Health Improvement was established to monitor and help improve the quality of health care provided by the NHS.

The terms of the Act enable the Secretary of State to require general medical practitioners, general dental practitioners, optometrists and pharmacists to hold approved indemnity cover (this was an area that the GOC had already reviewed).

Changes were made in an attempt to tackle fraud in the NHS. A civil penalty was created that could be imposed where a person fails to pay an NHS charge or claims a payment to which he is not entitled towards the cost of an NHS charge or service. Further knowingly making false representations to evade or gain a reduction or remission of, or a payment relating to, NHS charges became a criminal offence. It also becomes possible for a body corporate or an individual practitioner to be disqualified from providing ophthalmic services locally or if considered appropriate nationally.

The final element of this legislation that could impact on optometry is a change to the format of making Orders in Council regarding regulation of health care professionals. This would allow for the GOC to put forward changes that would otherwise require Parliamentary debate and inclusion within an Act of Parliament for the government to agree and introduce through SI.

Regional Variations in NHS Legislation with Respect to Ophthalmic Services

The foregoing section has dealt with legislation passed by parliament in London, and although there was until recently little variation in the regions these regulations apply specifically to England and Wales. During the development of the NHS there have been, for either environmental or political reasons, separate sets of regulations to cover Scotland and Northern Ireland. As devolution progresses separate regulations relating to health care have been implemented and for the first time Wales is able to regulate aspects of health care independent of parliament in London.

Scotland

Although separate legislation existed for the NHS in Scotland, for the most part the GOS provided has been the same as in England and Wales. The original legislative framework for the NHS in Scotland was set out in the National Health Service (Scotland) Act 1978. The most significant differences existed in the administrative structure and in the provision of services for remote areas.

Under the new devolved executive the 15 Health Board areas will remain and each will have a single unified NHS Board to replace the previous NHS Health Boards and NHS Trusts. Four main measures are planned to pull together the work of primary care, acute services and health improvement the different component parts of the local NHS system. These four principal measures are:

- making all parts of the local NHS system accountable through the new NHS Board
- introduction of a single Local Health Plan to ensure a more consistent and cohesive approach to planning
- a new performance and accountability framework
- revised financial arrangements.

The unified NHS Board will be a strategic body accountable to the Scottish Executive Health Department and to ministers responsible for planning and performance management and not normally day-to-day operational issues.

Advisory committees will still play an important role in the function of the boards and an optometric adviser has been appointed to the Scottish Executive.

The GOS have been arranged on behalf of the Health Boards by three joint ophthalmic committees and this is unlikely to change. It is the responsibility of these committees to establish the ophthalmic lists. The committees also have power to investigate breaches of NHS contracts either directly or via service committees. Corresponding to the areas of the joint ophthalmic committee there is a provision for the recognition of three joint area optical committees. As in England, practitioner representatives form area optical committees that correspond to the LOCs of England. These area optical committees are set up for each of the health board areas.

The second major difference between the service provided is with respect to remote areas where patients may not be able to visit a practitioner without either an excessive journey or an overnight stay. In such cases it has been possible for the joint ophthalmic committee to make special arrangements. This is likely to continue although the island boards are to be the subject of a separate review to identify the most suitable approach to take.

The devolution of power to Scotland has impacted already on the way the NHS develops in the future.

Northern Ireland

As with Scotland, the major differences between the ophthalmic services of Northern Ireland and those of England lie in the administrative structure, headed by the Northern Ireland Department of Health and Social Services. The hospitals and practitioner services are administered by four Health and Social Services Boards under the authority of that department. The GOS are established by the Health and Social Services Boards but are administered in part by a Central Services Agency, the functions of which are to maintain the ophthalmic lists and to pay fees and reimbursements to ophthalmic medical practitioners, ophthalmic opticians and dispensing opticians. The agency itself is advised and assisted by the Ophthalmic Committee and an Ophthalmic Officer/Adviser.

The other major difference in the ophthalmic services relates to the provision of services to schoolchildren. This section provides for medical practitioners to visit schools, test sight and give a prescription which is to be taken to either an optometrist or a dispensing optician registered to offer GOS.

As Northern Ireland also has its own devolved government it is likely that legislation on health care issues will develop differently to those in the other constituent regions of the UK.

Wales

The national Assembly for Wales (Transfer of Functions) Order 1999 SI 1999/672 has moved many of the functions of the Secretary of State in relation to the NHS to the National Assembly for Wales. Already it is apparent that there are developments within Wales that will allow ophthalmic services to be provided in a different format. While such changes are as yet embryonic once introduced it will effectively provide a different service for those in Wales compared to patients in England.

Wales has established Local Health Groups (equivalent to Primary Care Groups/Trusts in England) to act as the providers of primary care. Unlike England an optometrist is appointed to the management of the group by right. There are also provisions in place to remove HAs reducing the administrative tier structure and providing a closer link with practitioners and patients. It is still early to predict the outcome but health is being treated as a priority by the new assembly.

4

The National Health Service – Terms of Service

For most practitioners at least half of their time will be spent working with patients who qualify for examination under the National Health Service (NHS). Few if any practices currently survive by seeing private patients exclusively although this may change in the future if optometry follows the route of dentistry in the UK. Figures for the year to April 2000 indicated that the split of NHS to private examinations is 57/43 (Optics at a Glance FODO).

In order to provide NHS examinations optometrists, ophthalmic medical practitioners and bodies corporate must first register with the Health Authority (HA) responsible for the location in which they intend to offer the service. Inclusion on a HA's list of providers (ophthalmic list) automatically seals a contract with that HA under which the contractor agrees to abide by the 'terms of service' for the provision of NHS services. Failure to comply may result in legal action. The exception to this is for domiciliary providers who need to register with either the HA in which their office is registered or with each HA in which they provide services.

What is the Contract?

Essentially the contract is for the HA to make payments to a listed contractor for the delivery of services provided within the scope of the NHS. In return for such payments the contractor agrees to abide by the National Health Service (General Ophthalmic Services) Regulations 1986 (Statutory Instrument (SI) 1986/975) and subsequent amendments. As a result patients are provided with local ophthalmic services of set standard and the hospital eye service (I IES) is not inundated with patients seeking eye examinations.

What Does the Contract Entail?

The requirements of the contract include both clinical and non-clinical aspects of practice and can be broken down into the following sub-headings:

- registration
- establishing patient eligibility for GOS
- changes to contract
- general facilities
- testing of sight
- records
- informing and referral
- deputies and employees

- complaints
- NHS action.

These are considered in more detail below.

Registration

To be entered onto the appropriate ophthalmic list an individual or body corporate must undertake to provide General Ophthalmic Services (GOS) and to comply with the terms of service. Any application must contain:

- the name of the person or body corporate entitled to be included
- the address of all places in the HA's locality at which they undertake to provide GOS
- particulars of the days and hours at which services will normally be available
- the names of all other ophthalmic medical practitioners (OMPs) or optometrists who regularly provide GOS at the same addresses.

Establishing patient eligibility for GOS

An eligible person wishing to have a NHS sight test may apply to any contractor who appears on a HA's ophthalmic list. However, before any service is provided, the contractor must satisfy him/herself that a sight test is necessary and that the individual is entitled to a NHS test. Where a patient is claiming eligibility the optometrist has to verify that evidence has been produced supporting eligibility. If no evidence is available the contractor has to indicate this on the GOS form. The contractor must then ensure that the required patient information and approximate date of the last sight test are inserted onto the NHS sight test form. The terms of service do not specify that the exact date of the last sight test must be included.

Eligibility for a NHS test is defined within SI 1986/975 and subsequent amendments as relating to persons:

1 Under the age of 16 years.
2 Under the age of 19 years and receiving qualifying full-time education. The cut-off point for educational eligibility in the summer term for those changing educational activities has been agreed as the September following the end of the normal summer term. This means that students continuing in education will state their last school as the educational establishment until they confirm their place for the next academic year.
3 Over 60 years of age.
4 Requiring to wear complex lenses.
5 Registered blind or partially sighted under Section 29 of the National Assistance Act 1948.
6 Diagnosed as suffering from diabetes or glaucoma. This category includes:
   (a) patients who previously have suffered from glaucoma but the condition is considered to be treated

(b) patients with high intra-ocular pressure who have been advised by their ophthalmologist that they are at risk of glaucoma even though it is not currently present.

7 Aged 40 or over and the parent, brother, sister or child of a person who has been diagnosed as suffering from glaucoma.

8 Considered having resources less than, or equal to, his/her requirements. To define this more precisely people with the following status are considered to fall within this category:

(a) in receipt of income support

(b) a member of the same family as a person who is in receipt of income support

(c) in receipt of working families' tax credit

(d) a member of the same family as a person who is in receipt of working families' tax credit

(e) in receipt of a disabled persons' tax credit (at maximum rate, or reduced by £70.00 or less)

(f) a member of the same family as a person in category (e)

(g) in receipt of an income-based job seekers allowance

(h) a member of the same family as a person who is in receipt of an income-based job seekers allowance

(i) patients who are named on a valid NHS low income scheme certificate that may be HC2 (entitling the named persons to an NHS sight test and full voucher values) or HC3 which is for limited help.

To help further define 'family' eligibility the term is given the meaning provided by the Social Security Contributions and Benefits Act 1992 except for cases (i) and (j) where it has the meaning given by the Jobseekers Act 1995!

A contractor is required to check wherever possible the eligibility of a patient for exemption from charges. This requires a patient to provide evidence of entitlement and where appropriate the evidence (such as entitlement number, general practitioner (GP) details, etc.) should be included on the NHS form. A practitioner should have sight of exemption certificates HC2 or HC3 and where appropriate other documentary proof of exemption. Where exemption is on age grounds evidence of date of birth should be provided. If such evidence is not available then the appropriate roundel on the GOS form must be marked with an X. Once evidence on the basis of age has been shown it is not necessary for the practitioner to demand such evidence at each subsequent visit and it is therefore important to note on the record card when evidence is seen.

The terms of service further define who may sign a form on behalf of a patient. Normally this will be a parent or guardian or person who has care for the individual. The contractor MUST NOT sign the form on behalf of the patient. A separate signature space is provided on the GOS form for a signature on behalf of the patient.

Changes to contract

Practitioners have a duty to keep up to date with changes in Health Service arrangements. There are moves for this to become electronic via the Department of Health web-site. It is normally the responsibility of the HA to distribute relevant documentation by sending it to any address notified by the practitioner. As practitioners are required to notify the HA of all changes in address this should not be a problem. However, should the practitioner fail to keep the HA informed and details of a change in the terms of service are sent out by the HA but not received, the practitioner will be considered at fault if he/she fails to comply. It is essential therefore for the contractor to ensure all address changes be notified. Ignorance through non-receipt due to failure to notify a change of address is not a defence.

A contractor wishing to withdraw from the list needs to give written notice and normally will be withdrawn at the expiration of 3 months. In the case of a contractor dying or otherwise ceasing to be an OMP or optometrist the name will be withdrawn 6 months after services cease to be provided.

General facilities

A contractor can only provide GOS at an address that is included in his/her entry in the ophthalmic list or at the residential address of a patient eligible for a domiciliary visit or at certain specified day centres or residential homes appearing on the lists of an HA. If services are to be provided at another location an application has to be made to the HA for the new address to be included in the ophthalmic list.

Proper and sufficient waiting and consulting room accommodation and suitable equipment for provision of GOS must be provided. No criteria are available to define proper, suitable and sufficient. However, it is a requirement that a contractor must admit an authorized officer of the HA who has made a written request to inspect accommodation or equipment. The terms of the contract require the contractor to admit an authorized officer at all reasonable times.

Also part of the terms of service is a requirement to display prominently a notice and leaflet supplied or approved by the HA indicating the NHS' services available and NHS payments and charges.

Testing of sight

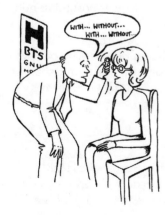

The NHS require a contractor who is listed as providing GOS to test the sight of any eligible patient to determine whether the patient needs to wear or use an optical appliance and in so doing to comply with the requirements of the Opticians Act 1989. Any prescription issued must be in the form recommended in Appendix A to the BS 3521:1962 and must comply with any requirements issued by the Secretary of State. There have been queries recently as to whether a prescription can be issued to a patient on a form other than the NHS produced form. The regulations do not specify that the NHS form must be used for issue of a prescription to a patient however any prescription must comply with the requirements of the Opticians Act 1989.

The Sight Testing (Examination and Prescription) (No. 2) Regulations 1989 (SI 1989/1230) also state that any prescription provided in fulfilment of the duty imposed by the Opticians Act must include:

1 details of the lenses prescribed
2 date of testing of sight

3 name and address of the patient and if under 16 date of birth
4 name and practice address of optometrist who carried out testing of sight
5 a statement of no change if there is no prescription change or an insignifi-cant prescription change.

Records

As may be expected a contractor agrees to keep a proper record concern-ing each patient to whom GOS are provided. The record must give appropriate details of the testing of sight. It is also a requirement that all such records are maintained for a period of 7 years. Furthermore, if required, the contractor must produce the record for any authorized officer within a specified period that will not be less than 14 days. In the current climate of fraud allegations it is even more crucial that records are well maintained and meet the requirements of the terms of service.

Informing and referral

Under the terms of service a contractor should inform the patient's GP where:

- on examination a patient shows signs of injury, disease or abnormality in the eye or elsewhere which may require medical treatment
- a satisfactory standard of vision is not achieved even when using corrective lenses
- a patient diagnosed as diabetic is examined
- a patient diagnosed as suffering from glaucoma is examined.

These NHS regulations run in parallel with the GOC regulations (see Chapter 5) but unlike the GOC rules are only relevant to patients seen within the GOS.

Deputies and employees

The contract specifies that in the case of deputies an OMP may arrange for sight to be tested on his/her behalf by another OMP. Similarly an optometrist may arrange for sight to be tested on his/her behalf by another optometrist. It is the responsibility of the contractor to notify the HA if the arrangement becomes regular and to ensure the inclusion of the deputy in the ophthalmic list. A contractor is responsible for all acts and omissions of a deputy acting on his behalf.

When employing a deputy an OMP can only employ another OMP and an optometrist another optometrist or a person acting under continuous personal supervision who is authorized to test sight.

Complaints

Recent changes to the terms of service have added a requirement for con-tractors to comply with a complaints procedure to deal with any complaints by or on behalf of patients or former patients. This whole area is discussed in Chapter 6.

NHS action

The effect of applying for and being included in the ophthalmic list is to accept the terms of service and become a contractor with the HA. Failure to comply would be considered as a breach of the contract. There are a number of actions open to an HA depending on the severity of the breach. Recently the profession has seen a series of investigations into alleged fraud. Allegations have been made, for example, of submitting forms for non-existent patients or for falsely claiming for domiciliary visits. Such cases may be taken by the HA to the Courts.

In clinical cases (such as failure to complete a satisfactory examination) it is possible for the HA to establish a process of investigation and panel review. This may be followed by full Tribunal Hearings and these are discussed in Chapter 6.

Key points 1: Non-clinical contractual requirements

1 To provide adequate waiting and consulting space
2 To notify the HA of changes of address
3 To check patient eligibility for GOS
4 To display required posters and leaflets
5 To complete relevant forms accurately

Key points 2: Clinical contractual requirements

1 To have adequate equipment available to provide NHS ophthalmic services
2 To test sight as defined by the Opticians Act
3 To issue a valid prescription as required
4 To inform the GP as specified
5 To keep proper records for a minimum of 7 years

The National Health Service General Ophthalmic Services

The terms of service for an optometrist registering to provide National Health Service (NHS) optometric services within a Health Authority (HA) appear in Chapter 4. In addition to the regulations found within terms of service there are other General Ophthalmic Services (GOS) regulations that apply to practice. A guide to these together with a reference to the source documents is given below.

Frequency of Eye Examinations

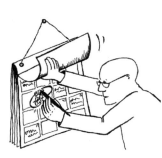

Note FPN 713 issued in October 1997 states 'it is for optometrists and ophthalmic medical practitioners (OMPs) to decide how frequently a patient's sight needs testing'. It then goes on to state that in the view of the Department of Health adult patients with refractive errors but no under-lying disease or risk factors should not need tests more often than every 2 years. This statement however has not been accepted as valid by the profession and several schemes to identify frequency of testing needs have been produced. It has been particularly difficult to reach agreement on the frequency of sight testing for children with visual problems. Currently the professional bodies are working together to produce guidance. Guidance on this issue has also been published for Northern Ireland and Scotland.

Whatever the outcome it is essential that good case records are maintained to support any decisions to provide early re-testing.

Display of Notices

At each premises at which a contractor provides GOS an HA approved notice and leaflet must be prominently displayed indicating the services available under the GOS and terms of eligibility for such services (SI 1996/705).

Information must be provided about the complaints procedure oper-ated within the practice, the details should include details of the person nominated within the practice to investigate and deal with complaints (SI 1996/705).

Small Frame Supplement

Introduced in 1997 this additional payment was intended to cover the situ-ation in which a non-standard frame and lenses had to be produced at additional cost in which the datum centres were not more than 56 mm apart (or box centre distances of not more than 55 mm). The requirements were however changed in HSC 1999/051 when small frames became available as standards from stock. The new definition states 'small glasses means glasses for a child under 7 years who needs a custom made or a stock spectacle frame which requires extensive adaptation to ensure an accurate fit and has a boxed centre of no more than 55 mm. For this purpose boxed centre is to be construed in accordance with Part 1 of BS 3521/91 (terms relating to optics and spectacle frames) published by the BSI'.

Examples of extensive adaptations are given as:

- reductions or increases in the length of sides
- manipulations to reduce or increase the bridge width which cannot be achieved solely by adjustment of the pads
- lenses with a high, positive spherical power worked to minimum substance (either by the practice or a wholesale supplier).

Where exceptionally a patient of 7 or over requires small glasses the HA should be consulted (NHS (Optical Charges and Payments) Regulations 1997, SI 1999/609 and HSC 1999/051).

Tinted Lenses

Under the GOS a tint should only be prescribed if it is judged to be clinically necessary, tints for cosmetic purposes are not available under the GOS. It is acceptable to provide a photochromic tint where appropriate and clinically necessary as specified in HSC 1999/051. Anti-reflection coatings and ultraviolet (UV) blocking tints cannot normally be supplied under the terms of the GOS. For some patients undergoing dermatological treatment where there may be a risk to the eyes from UV light it would be possible to provide a UV filter under the Hospital Eye Service (HES) regulations. Plano-tinted spectacles for assistance in dealing with children with dyslexia are not covered within the GOS regulations (FPN 713 and HSC 1999/051).

Non-tolerance

If a second eye test is undertaken due to an intolerance of the prescription by the patient then any new GOS form submitted should be annotated 're-test/non-tolerance'. Having completed the test a new voucher cannot be issued without the prior approval of the HA. If authority is given by telephone then the Voucher should be annotated with the name of the person authorizing and the date on which authority was given (FPN 713).

Completing Form GOS 1

Once eligibility for a sight test has been demonstrated the details on the form should be duly completed. It is not necessary for the patient to complete the details but it is necessary for the patient to sign the form to confirm that the details are correct (SI 1997/818).

Altering Prescriptions

Transposition

All prescriptions issued under the GOS should be written in the highest spherical power to provide for the optimum patient voucher value. If as a supplier a prescription is received that is not in this form then it can be amended on the voucher and then the amendments initialled and annotated FPN : 713 (FPN 713).

In the case of a HES (P) form no changes can be made to the form in which the prescription is written even if transposition would prove an advantage to the patient by increasing the value of the voucher.

Back vertex distance changes

Where it is found necessary to amend a voucher prescription to take account of back vertex distance (BVD) then the supplier should initial the changes and add 'BVD change'. If however amending the prescription takes it to a higher voucher band then the prescribers authority to make the amendment is required. It would be necessary for the prescriber to amend and initial the voucher or to send a note or fax authorizing the change (FPN 713).

Complex Lenses

A complex lens is defined as a lens with a power in any one meridian of ±10 dioptres (D) or a prism controlled bifocal lens. Any patient requiring a complex lens is entitled to a NHS sight test and they may also be issued with a complex lens voucher unless they are entitled to a spectacle voucher on income grounds in which case they cannot receive the additional amount for a complex lens. A patient entitled to a complex lens voucher would also be entitled to supplements for tints, prisms or small frames.

If a patient, previously requiring a complex lens is found during an NHS sight test to no longer require a complex lens he/she would still be eligible to receive an NHS sight test on this one occasion even though he/she does not meet the eligibility requirement (FPN 713).

Small Prescription Changes

Where a sight test results in a small prescription change that is considered clinically insignificant a voucher should not be issued other than when spectacles are to be replaced for fair wear and tear (FPN 713).

Lifetime of a Prescription

The maximum lifetime of a prescription is 2 years and spectacles should not normally be made up to a prescription that is more than 2 years old (HSC 1999/051 and SI 1984/1778).

Issuing of a Voucher

A voucher should be issued at the time of the NHS sight test to all those eligible. The patient should sign Part 1 of the form GOS 3 at this time to confirm eligibility. The patient may take the voucher to any supplier legally able to provide them with an optical appliance. The patient should sign Part 2 of the form GOS 3 upon receipt of spectacles (FPN 713).

Lifetime of a Voucher

Once issued, unless a shorter time is indicated, a voucher has a lifetime of 2 years to bring it in line with the maximum life of a prescription. Where a patient appears to have lost a voucher the HA can authorize a practice to issue another once it is confirmed that the voucher has not already been used. This authorization to issue a second voucher can be given to a practice that did not issue the original voucher. Any voucher issued in this way should be annotated with the name of the person at the HA giving authority and should carry the date on which the replacement was issued (SI 1999/609 and HSC 1999/051).

Submission of Vouchers

Vouchers for sight testing (GOS 1) should be submitted to the appropriate HA for payment within three months of the date on which the sight test took place. Vouchers for the supply of optical appliances or repair or replacement should be submitted within 3 months of the date on which the appliance was supplied, repaired or replaced (SI 1997/819).

Change of Eligibility Status

If a patient can show evidence of NHS eligibility following a private sight test and before ordering spectacles it is not necessary to undergo a second test. Instead the supplier should complete a GOS 3 form and copy over the details of the private prescription (HSG (97)48 and FPN 706).

Spare Pairs of Spectacles and Repairs and Replacements

No patient has ever been automatically entitled to a spare pair of glasses of the same prescription. Exceptionally – for example, where a child with a disabling illness is breaking glasses with such frequency that education is being disrupted – permission may be sought from the HA to allow supply of a second pair. In the case of permission for a second pair claims should be submitted on form GOS 5/GOS 3 and the form annotated with the name of the person at the HA who gave authority.

Where a spare pair has been issued under these arrangements the patient is entitled to have either pair replaced or repaired provided that they are children or that the HA has accepted the loss/breakage is due to illness. You should not repair or replace an adult's spectacles until the HA is satisfied that the breakage or loss was due to illness. In very exceptional circumstances of major hardship an HA may consider replacement of stolen or broken spectacles without which the patient would have extreme difficulty in working (FPN 706 and FPN 713).

In the case of supply of an appliance by a hospital to a child repairs can be carried out and claims made on a GOS 4 form. Where an adult is supplied with an appliance through the HES they should be advised to consult the hospital in the case of loss or breakage (FPN 713).

If a patient has been tested and no change made to spectacles but spectacles are then broken shortly after the test, where the optometrist judges that there was unlikely to have been any change in prescription, a voucher could be issued on the grounds of fair wear and tear without a further examination (SI 1999/609 and FPN 713).

High Reading Additions

To assist patients who may otherwise seek to apply for a low vision aid the voucher appropriate to bifocal spectacles is to be determined by the power of the reading add when it is more than 4.00 D more powerful than the distance prescription. For all other bifocal prescriptions the voucher value is determined solely by the power of the distance segment (HSC 1999/051).

Payments by Instalment

If a patient opts to buy glasses by instalment but subsequently establishes eligibility for a refund of a voucher value no refund will be made until such time as the patient has paid instalments equivalent to the voucher value (SI 1999/609 and HSC 1999/051).

Patient Refunds

A patient applying for a refund must establish their eligibility within three months of the date on which they paid for the glasses or, in the case of payment by instalment made the first payment (SI 1999/609, FPN 706 and HSC 1999/051).

Contact Lenses

A patient may put the spectacle voucher towards the purchase of contact lenses but the prescription written for spectacles should not be amended. Where the contact lens prescription is in a higher or lower band than that for the spectacles the voucher value appropriate to the spectacles should be issued. A voucher for replacement of 'durable' contact lenses can be issued on the basis of fair wear and tear if an optometrist judges them to be unserviceable. Within the terms of the GOS contact lenses will be considered to be disposable if they require replacement at 6-monthly intervals or less. A voucher should not be issued for supply of further disposable contact lenses on the grounds of fair wear and tear and may only be issued on the basis of a change of prescription at a valid re-examination (FPN 713).

Where a patient loses or breaks a contact lens which is not defined as disposable within the GOS and is eligible for replacement (i.e. a child or an adult judged by the HA to have lost or broken the lens through illness) a voucher for replacement spectacles should be issued. If the patient wishes this voucher can be put towards the cost of a replacement contact lens.

Varifocals

If a patient is supplied with varifocals as an alternative to bifocals then a voucher may be issued and the value claimed is as if bifocals had been supplied (FPN 713).

Eligibility for a NHS Sight Test Relating to Glaucoma

Anyone undergoing treatment for glaucoma and anyone who has undergone surgery for glaucoma is entitled to a NHS sight test.

Any patient who has been referred to the ophthalmology department with raised intra-ocular pressure (IOP) and suspect glaucoma and found clear but advised by the ophthalmologist to seek regular monitoring because they are at risk of glaucoma may be treated as eligible for NHS sight tests.

Parents, siblings and children of patients in the above categories who are over 40 years of age are eligible for NHS sight tests (FPN 713 and SI 1999/693).

Eligibility for a NHS Sight Test due to Diabetes

Once diagnosed patients suffering from diabetes are always likely to be at risk of diabetic eye changes and therefore should continue to be eligible for GOS. It is a requirement of the terms of service to report findings to the GP following every examination of a person claiming NHS eligibility due to the presence of diabetes.

Overseas Visitors' Eligibility to Receive NHS GOS

Eligibility for NHS treatment in the UK relates to whether a person is ordinarily resident in the UK and not to nationality, payment of National Insurance contributions or taxes. The courts have decided that a person is regarded as 'ordinarily resident' in the UK if he or she is lawfully living in the UK voluntarily and for a settled purpose as part of the regular order of his or her life for the time being. It is considered unlikely that anyone coming to live in the UK, intending to stay for less than 6 months will fulfil the criteria. A refugee given leave to remain in the UK or who is in the UK awaiting the result of an application to remain in the UK should be regarded as ordinarily resident. If a patient's chargeable status is not clear private charges should be paid and the patient given a receipt and advised to seek clarification and if appropriate a refund from the NHS (HSC 1999/018).

Student Eligibility for GOS on Age Grounds

Students leaving school and continuing education by starting at a university or college and who would be eligible for GOS on age grounds remain eligible between leaving school and starting university or college provided that they do not intend taking time out. Time out is considered as being when they do not intend to leave school and start further/higher education in the same calendar year. If they have left school they should enter in the appropriate section of the GOS forms, the name of the university or the college they are due to attend.

Reglazing Spectacles

Where a patient whose prescription has changed opts to use an existing frame for reglazing, Form GOS 5/GOS 3 should be completed and the appropriate voucher value or the cost of the reglaze, whichever is lower, should be claimed. If only one lens is to be reglazed a claim for the voucher value or the private charge for one lens whichever is lower can be submitted. There are no 'half' vouchers and the full voucher value will be due if the normal private retail price for the supply and fitting of one lens exceeds the voucher value.

Where a prescription has changed in one eye only but the patient requests a new frame the appropriate voucher value or the cost of supply of the new spectacles, whichever is the lower, should be claimed (FPN 713).

Point of Service Checks

Introduced in February 2001 a point of service check on eligibility must be carried out when a patient applies for a sight test on the NHS or a voucher for supply of an optical appliance is accepted. Where no evidence is available the GOS form should be marked accordingly (GOS circular January 2001).

Domiciliary Visits

When carrying out a domiciliary visit the patient must indicate the health problems that prevent them from attending a practice. The patient or the carer will need to certify that they have requested a domiciliary visit, because of inability to leave home, by completing the appropriate box on the GOS form.

Mobile practices are required to register with the home HA where the business offices are situated and the host HA where they intend to provide domiciliary service.

Domiciliary Services to day centres are limited to those that provide for:

- patients with disabilities who would otherwise require a sight test at home
- children with special needs attending non-residential schools
- members of ethnic communities unaccustomed to using mainstream health care facilities and who would be best served by receiving care in their community surroundings
- genuinely homeless people of no fixed abode who are unlikely to be able to access services in a community practice.

Even when day centres fall within these categories patients must be non-ambulant or incapable of accessing community optical practices without undue difficulty (GOS circular January 2001).

6

Complaints and National Health Service Tribunals

The NHS terms of service for ophthalmic services (National Health Service (General Ophthalmic Services (GOS)) Regulations 1986 SI 1986 No. 975) were reviewed in Chapter 4. The aim of this chapter is to outline the processes and most likely sources of action for an alleged breach of the NHS contract. In practice there are two main processes that can be brought into play when practitioners fall down in their NHS role. The first process is patient driven and the second process is Health Authority (HA) driven.

The terms of service require a practice to have in place a complaint procedure that acts as the first step in dealing with a patient complaint. This allows minor disagreements to be dealt with effectively within practice and avoids intervention by an HA. A new procedure introduced in April 1996 by replacing the formal handling of complaints by the statutory (service committee) system and separating complaint handling from disciplinary procedures further emphasized the concept of practice-based responsibility for dealing with complaints (SI 1996/705). The aim of the new system is to provide an opportunity for practices to recognize and change any problem areas and improve services. A booklet on the complaint procedures is available to patients through the NHS and helps them to understand how to proceed.

A second aspect of terms of service is to require optometrists and bodies corporate to meet specific standards and provide services as agreed. It is the responsibility of the HA to monitor the standards of service provision in their area. Should a practitioner or body corporate not meet the required standard or breach the terms of service the HA will take appropriate action.

Patient Complaint Procedures

National criteria

When introducing the concept of practice-based complaint or 'local resolution' procedures, the NHS issued details of agreed criteria. Providing these are met implementation of the procedures is flexible and can be adapted to fit the needs of individual practices.

The basic criteria are:

- the complaint procedure should be managed entirely within the practice
- everyone working within the practice should understand the system
- one person within the practice should be nominated to administer the procedure
- publicity should be given to the procedure within the practice

- complaints should normally be acknowledged within 2 working days
- an explanation should normally be provided within 10 working days.

Although set up as part of the NHS terms of service the complaints procedure is not restricted to NHS issues. The HA will only become involved:

- at the request of a practice
- if procedures do not meet the agreed criteria
- when a satisfactory outcome cannot otherwise be achieved.

Meeting the national criteria

For the procedure to work effectively and to avoid HA involvement it is essential for a practice to set up a system that meets both the national criteria and its own circumstances.

The first stage in establishing a system involves discussion of the aims and the benefits with all members of staff. It is essential that everyone involved co-operates, uses the system positively and understands the value of resolving a problem 'in house' without the involvement of outside agencies. Once the initial discussion is completed one person within the practice should be nominated to administer the procedure. It helps if the nominated individual is committed to the process!

Publicity for the procedure is necessary although there have been arguments to the effect that promoting the existence of the procedure could encourage complaints. There does not appear to be any evidence for this at this stage. The criteria require a waiting area poster to be displayed and written information to be available detailing the complaint procedure within the practice. The Department of Health can provide a generic poster and leaflets.

Information provided to the patient should:

- identify the contact individual within the practice
- outline the process after first contact is made
- identify who will contact them as the next stage
- indicate time scales for events
- offer possible outcomes for the procedure
- provide details of how to access HA complaint procedures.

Any patient who feels unable to deal with their practitioner directly can approach the HA with a complaint. The HA may then act as intermediary between practice and patient and where appropriate offer a conciliation service.

Record keeping

It is advisable to keep accurate practice records of *all* complaints made, investigations carried out and outcomes. This provides a review process to analyse any recurring problems and support practice development and improvement in quality of service. Records also provide evidence of action taken should the complaint not be resolved within the practice.

Records should include copies of all correspondence, notes of all telephone conversations and meetings including dates, times and those involved, and information on action taken. It is important that these notes are kept separate from the clinical records of a patient.

The records are practice property and will not be requested by the HA should further action occur. However, if a request is made the records should be provided for the person complaining. There is an apparent conflict here in that the records could be made available to an HA by a patient lodging a complaint.

The new complaints procedures have been in place since 1 April 1996 and therefore should be well established. The types of complaint will range from dissatisfaction with quality of product or service to queries on price or delivery times. In some cases the complaints may relate to clinical competence, for example, failure to carry out an adequate examination or to detect a condition. As there are no financial costs for the patient, the procedure could be used as a means of testing the validity of a case prior to civil action.

Keeping control

In any complaint situation it is important to remember:

- keep as calm as possible
- try to keep the patient as calm as possible
- if possible move to a private area for discussion
- listen carefully to the complaint and try to understand the patient's view
- establish the facts and understand the complaint
- if unsure of your position do not make hasty decisions – offer to review the details of the complaint and get back to the patient
- avoid admitting liability
- establish what action the patient is seeking
- in many cases it will be more cost-effective, without admitting liability, to change a product or offer a goodwill refund than to have a protracted argument
- if you do not settle the issue it will go to the HA.

Beyond Local Resolution

The intention is that all complaints should be dealt with in the above process but inevitably there are some cases where the two parties are unable to agree on facts, actions, outcomes or settlement and the process then moves on. The second phase of the procedure is termed 'independent review' and involves the senior member of staff within the HA with responsibility for managing complaints and a non-executive director of the Authority, known as a Convenor. The two review all submissions and decide on the most appropriate route for the complaint. There are five likely options should a complaint reach this second phase:

- complaint is referred back to the practice if it is felt more could be achieved
- conciliation is arranged to try to resolve the issue without further process

- an independent review panel is established to look at the complaint
- no further action is taken where it appears everything possible has been done
- the complainant is advised of their right to approach the Health Ombudsman.

Review panels

When considering the review panel option the Convenor will be assisted by an independent lay Chairperson nominated by the Secretary of State for Health. At this point clinical advice will be available to the Convenor from optometrists based outside the HA's area and nominated by Local Optical Committees (LOCs) or the Professional Body (College of Optometry).

Although any complaint can progress to the second phase it is likely that only the more serious such as failure to complete a satisfactory examination, provision of inadequate spectacle correction or failure to refer appropriately will be considered for a review panel assessment.

It is important to note that the review panel has no disciplinary function but is established to try to resolve the complaint as constructively as possible. There is no obligation on the panel to engage in lengthy evidence gathering or to hold formal hearings.

A review panel consists of three people:

- an independent lay Chairperson
- the Convenor
- a second lay member appointed by the Secretary of State for Health.

If the complaint to be considered is clinical in nature the panel would be supported by two independent optometrists nominated by LOCs. The role of these independent optometrists is to advise and to make a report on the clinical and technical facts to the panel.

After due consideration of all the information available the panel reports to the person complaining and to the practice involved and may make comments about service improvements. The review panel sends a copy of the report to the relevant department at the HA. No recommendations about disciplinary action are included and it is left to the HA to decide if any further action is appropriate.

Further appeal

If the complainant is still dissatisfied after the report from the review panel or if a review panel was not set up, there is an opportunity for a further process. This final stage involves the Health Service Commissioner (Ombudsman). Changes introduced in 1996 allow the Ombudsman to consider clinical matters where appropriate and it is for the Ombudsman after receiving clinical advice where necessary to decide on whether further investigation is warranted.

It can be seen from the above that any complaints process that extends beyond the local resolution, in addition to causing personal strain, is likely to involve considerable practitioner time. It is therefore always advisable to resolve matters within the practice if at all possible.

Health Authority Action

The disciplinary process

While the patient-driven complaint procedure and independent review panel report can result in an HA disciplinary process it is possible for the HA to initiate its own disciplinary process. Action is taken where it is considered that a practitioner has failed to comply with the terms of service or where an HA considers that an overpayment has been made to a practitioner but the practitioner does not admit to the overpayment. The procedures for the investigation of such matters and subsequent disciplinary process are lengthy. For those interested they can be found in the National Health Service (Service Committees and Tribunal) Regulation 1992 (b), the National Health Service (Service Committees and Tribunal) Amendment Regulations 1995 and the National Health Service (Service Committees and Tribunal) Amendment Regulations 1996.

In essence an HA refers any such matter for disciplinary investigation to another, unlinked, HA. It is then for the relevant committee of the HA receiving the referral to proceed and to produce a report on the matter. The original referring HA then considers the report and appropriate actions.

Normally there are two potential outcomes to an HA consideration:

- no further action should be taken
- the practitioner is found to have failed to comply with the terms of service.

In the latter case the following penalties may be imposed:

- determine a financial penalty to be recovered from the practitioner
- warn the practitioner to comply more closely with the terms of service
- both of the above.

The ultimate sanction, however, for persistent breach of terms of service would be refusal by the HA to accept a practitioner on their list.

Audit procedures

There is a further non-clinical way for practitioners to become involved in HA proceedings and one that is currently very topical. All HAs are required to monitor their service and therefore have sampling procedures for checking submitted claims. Standard figures on prescribing of prisms or tints are produced locally and used as a performance indicator for monitoring prescribing habits amongst practitioners. Furthermore regular sampling checks are made on the validity of claims for NHS exemption of eye examination charges and dispensing claims. Recently these processes have led to investigation into fraud by practitioners within the GOS.

It is inevitable that occasional errors will occur in forms submitted or that some practitioners by virtue of expertise or locality will prescribe differently to the normal and this is accepted. Recently, however, there have been allegations of systematic, calculated attempts to defraud the health service. The methods used allegedly include:

- claiming too frequently for examinations
- claiming for deceased patients
- claiming for provision of a tint when no tint was provided
- claiming for a domiciliary visit when such a visit was not required.

In such cases the HA after consideration of the evidence may consider this to be more serious than a breach of the terms of service. This can result in a criminal investigation with evidence passed to the police for investigation and action.

Do you comply?

It is advisable to review your own complaint procedures. In registering with an HA to provide GOS every optometrist enters into a contract and agrees to abide by the terms of service. As discussed in Chapter 4 this means establishing a complaint procedure and agreeing to the procedures outlined above – ignorance is no defence!

Optical Consumer Complaints Service

Following the review of UK optical services by the optical service audit committee (OSAC) one of the recommendations was to establish an independent complaint service. This service was intended to cover all aspects of optical services and goods provided by registered optometrists and dispensing opticians. The result was the establishment of the optical consumer complaints service (OCCS) in 1993. Funding has been an issue since its start with the Association of British Dispensing Opticians (ABDO), Federation of Ophthalmic and Dispensing Opticians (FODO) and the Central LOC fund providing financial support but this is slowly resolving. OCCS was not set up as a disciplinary body but rather as a facilitator to try and achieve resolution of matters. It relies heavily on co-operation of practitioners. Where a practitioner fails to respond to a request from OCCS no further action can be taken other than to advise the patient on their rights and the processes remaining for them to pursue their complaint.

The service is open to anyone who is receiving or has received goods or services from an optical practice utilizing the services of an optometrist or a dispensing optician registered with the GOC. If someone other than the patient makes a complaint on the patients' behalf written authority from the patient is required before the complaint can be registered.

The level of contacts made is variable but appears to have settled at around 1100 per year and 50% of these are registered as a complaint for follow-up. When this is equated to the 15 million eye examinations carried out each year it can be seen that generally the profession works well.

Key points 1: General procedures for NHS complaints

1 Local resolution (patient driven)
2 Independent review (HA driven)
3 The Health Ombudsman (HA driven)

Key points 2: Independent review processes

1 Complaint referred back to the involved practice
2 Conciliation arranged
3 An independent review panel is initiated
4 A decision is made that no further action is considered necessary
5 The patient is advised of their rights to approach the Health Ombudsman

7

The Opticians Act

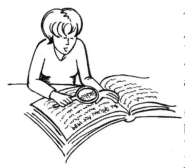

The primary statute relating to optical professional practice is the Opticians Act 1989. This was a consolidated Act based on the original Opticians Act 1958 but incorporating the various changes that had occurred in the intervening 30 years. As a consolidating Act there was no intention to introduce any additional changes to the legislation in place.

In spite of over 50 years of tremendous effort by the optical profession the original 1958 Opticians Act was not a government response to lobbying but the result of a Private Members Bill. Ronald Russell the Member for Wembley South presented his bill in 1957 and it received Royal Assent in July 1958. This Act completely changed optics and provided a firm footing for the separate development of the optometric and dispensing professions. Although there have been some substantial amendments, notably those of the Health and Social Security Act 1984, the basis of the Act with regard to 'promoting high standards of professional education and professional conduct among opticians' is retained.

Purposes of the Act

The main purposes of this Act were to establish:

1 a body with the function of promoting high standards of professional education and professional conduct among opticians and other functions assigned by or under the Act
2 and maintain registers of those qualified to provide sight testing, sight testing and dispensing and dispensing only
3 disciplinary procedures
4 restrictions on testing of sight, fitting of contact lenses, sale and supply of optical appliances and use of titles and descriptions
5 miscellaneous and supplementary matters relevant to the operation of the Act.

In addition to the main body of the Act a schedule was included specifying details of the General Optical Council (GOC) membership, the registrar role, powers of the GOC and powers of the Privy Council in relation to membership of the GOC.

The General Optical Council

The corner stone of the Opticians Act 1989 is the GOC. Established by the original 1958 Opticians Act this body has, amongst other duties, the task of maintaining standards. Currently the council is reviewing its structure and has proposed changes to both membership and committee format.

Essentially it will remain a mixture of professionals involved in eye care and lay individuals appointed by the Secretary of State for Health. The composition of the current GOC is determined by Part 1 of the Opticians Act 1989. Also set out are the main Committee structures and powers to enable the GOC to establish additional committees should this become necessary to enable the council to better perform its functions. The GOC is discussed in more detail in Chapter 8.

Registration and Training

Part 2 of the Act relating to Registration and Training of Opticians requires the GOC to maintain registers of suitably qualified individuals or corporate bodies carrying on business as either dispensing opticians or optometrists. In all there are currently three registers and two lists, the three registers dealing with individuals are of:

- optometrists who only test sight
- optometrists who both test sight and fit spectacles
- dispensing opticians.

To be included on any of the above registers individual applicants need to satisfy the GOC that they meet the requirements laid down in Section 8 of the Act. Essentially the requirements are for the individual to hold a recognized qualification and demonstrate evidence of 'adequate' experience although adequate is not defined. In addition to the above if the individual holds a recognized qualification gained outside of the UK they also need to satisfy the council they are of 'good character' before they are able to register.

The council keep under review qualifications offered outside of the UK and have established procedures for overseas optometrists wishing to register in the UK.

There is also a requirement that individuals do not appear in more than one register even if they hold qualifications entitling them to be included in more than one.

The enrolment of corporate bodies is also dealt with in Section 2 of the Act and the two lists maintained by the GOC are of:

- corporate bodies carrying on business as optometrists
- corporate bodies carrying on business as dispensing opticians.

For a corporate body to become enrolled they would need to comply with Section 9 of the Act. This specifies the requirements in terms of the type of business undertaken, directors, a grandfather clause and other relevant Acts of Parliament.

The basic information to be included in each entry in the lists is specified in the 1958 Act as:

1 names
2 addresses
3 qualifications.

The GOC is given the power under Section 10 to make rules concerning the form and keeping of the registers, amendments entitling registration and the fee to be charged for registration. Section 11 deals with publication of the lists and requires the GOC to publish a register as often as they think fit. Should a decision be made not to produce a register in any one year then a list of all alterations to the previously published list must be published.

The final sections of Part 2 of the Act relate to the recognition of suitable training institutions and qualifying examinations. The GOC has the role of determining whether the knowledge and skill provided for graduates are adequate for an institution to be considered for registration as an approved training institution. Where the GOC decides that an institution is not providing adequate training the institution has the right of appeal to the Privy Council who, if after consultation, think fit may reverse the decision. Visitors may be appointed by the GOC to attend institutions and qualifying examinations and produce reports of the findings of the visit as a way of maintaining standards. The GOC also make rules with regard to supervision of trainee optometrists.

The effect of Part 2 of the Act is to make it a criminal offence to gain registration by pretending to hold a qualification that would enable registration. It also lays down procedures for establishing and monitoring standards for initial training and qualification for all registered optometrists and dispensing opticians in practice in the UK.

Disciplinary Proceedings

Part 3 of the Act outlines the disciplinary proceedings and penalties for failing to meet the professional standards expected of a practitioner or body corporate. Failure may be:

1 not complying with regulations made under the terms of the Act (to include regulations made by the GOC or relevant Statutory Instruments, SIs)
2 by aiding or abetting others to break regulations
3 by acting in a way that the Disciplinary Committee of the GOC considers serious professional misconduct
4 by being convicted by any court in the UK of any criminal offence.

Three forms of disciplinary order are specified. These are:

1 *An erasure order:* under this outcome the name is removed from the relevant register and application has to be made for reinstatement (this cannot be made within 10 months of the erasure).
2 *A suspension order:* during the period of suspension (which may be up to a maximum of 1 year) the individual or corporate body involved will be treated as *not* being registered. At the end of the suspension period reinstatement is automatic.
3 *A penalty order:* a fine, the maximum value of which is specified in legislation and amended from time to time, may be imposed. This may be imposed in addition to either of the above two orders.

This part determines the options open to the GOC for dealing with lapses in professional standards by those appearing in any of the registers established under the Opticians Act. Such cases fall within the jurisdiction of the GOC and relate to fitness to practise.

Testing of Sight

It is Part 4 of the Act that has the greatest impact – this is the part relating to 'Restrictions on testing of sight, fitting of contact lenses, sale and supply of optical appliances and the use of titles and descriptions.' Offences within this section are considered criminal in nature and an action may be taken by any interested party through a court of law. Such actions may be taken by trading standards officers or the police for example, but normally it is the GOC who take action.

The very first section (24) states:

> ... a person who is not a registered medical practitioner or registered ophthalmic optician shall not test the sight of another person.

The definition of testing of sight has formed the basis of many discussions but in Section 36(2) of the Act is defined as:

> testing sight with the object of determining whether there is any and, if so, what defect of sight and of correcting, remedying or relieving any such defect of an anatomical or physiological nature by means of an optical appliance prescribed on the basis of the determination.

It is therefore a criminal offence for an individual who is not registered in one of the specified lists to carry out a sight test. The penalty for contravention is specified as a fine and a maximum level may be imposed for the fine (the current maximum penalty is £2500).

Section 25 sets out similar provisions for the fitting of contact lenses and again specifies those who are legally entitled to fit. Once again it is a criminal offence for an individual to fit contact lenses when they do not appear within the specified lists. Any case for contravention of this would be taken to court and if proven the individual would be liable to a fine up to the specified maximum level.

This part also imposes regulations regarding the duties that may be performed on sight testing by suitably qualified and registered practitioners. It is a legal requirement for the examination to be performed adequately. Immediately following the test a written statement should be issued indicating that an adequate examination was carried out and that referral is or is not required. In addition a signed written prescription or if no prescription is needed a note to that effect must also be issued.

Further regulations specify that it is an offence to require a patient, as a condition of undertaking the sight test, to purchase any optical appliance that may be necessary from a specified person. It is also an offence to require payment of a fee prior to the testing of sight of any individual and the fee is only payable where the required duties have been met.

Failure to comply with these requirements has in the past been considered by the GOC Disciplinary Committee as serious professional misconduct.

Sale and Supply of Optical Appliances

A further section (27) within Part 4 deals with the sale and supply of optical appliances. This was restricted to registered practitioners until the 1984 Health and Social Security Act that opened up the situation to allow for supply of spectacles by a much wider grouping. More recently the sale of 'ready readers' has also been allowed. The Opticians Act specifies that any sale or supply (other than for ready readers) must be effected against a written prescription issued by a registered medical practitioner or ophthalmic optician following a testing of sight by that individual. The written prescription must be within the time specified on the prescription with a maximum of 2 years as defined by SI 1984/1778.

It is a criminal offence to supply an optical appliance in contravention of the current legislation and on summary conviction an individual shall be liable to a fine.

Protection of Titles

The optical professions are further strengthened in this Act by the protection of specified titles for individuals and for bodies corporate. According to Section 28 of the Act the titles ophthalmic optician, optometrist, dispensing optician, registered optician or enrolled optician may only be used by those qualified for entry into the various registers. As a wider protection it is also a criminal offence to take or use any name, title, addition or description that falsely implies registration. Once again conviction for such an offence would result in the imposition of a fine.

Miscellaneous and Supplementary

A collection of 'tidying-up' sections form the final parts to the Act. In the main these relate to aspects of the GOC and cover the areas for which the GOC may make rules and the accounting procedures of the GOC. There are also sections relating to default powers of the Privy Council and the subordinate legislation procedure by which GOC rules come into force when approved by order of the Privy Council. These are normally exercisable by SI. A quorum of two is specified for the Privy Council to exercise powers under the Act.

The supplementary section is used to provide definitions for various terms that appear within the Act.

Schedule

The schedule to the Act provides details of the constitution and powers assigned to the GOC and these are discussed in Chapter 8.

Action under the Terms of the Act

As stated at the outset the Opticians Act forms the basis for the statutory regulation of the professions of optometry and dispensing optics in the UK. It is a mixture of criminal and professional statutes that apply to anyone involving themselves in the testing of sight and the supply of optical appliances. The GOC acts as the controller of standards and would be the body that would take action as necessary were failure to comply with the Act to be identified. Under the terms of the Act the GOC is also able to make supplementary legislation with regard to a series of issues and these will be dealt with in Chapter 9.

Has any action been taken over the past few years against individuals failing to comply with the Act itself? The answer is very definitely yes! Actions with regard to many facets of the Act have been pursued mainly through the GOC.

Lack of Registration

Action has been taken against individuals who have carried out eye examinations when they do not appear in the relevant register. The maximum fine that could be imposed by a court for each offence is £2500. In a case in 1997 brought by the GOC the individual concerned was found guilty of two charges relating to eye examinations. The Magistrates Court hearing the case found the individual guilty and imposed a fine of £250 for each charge and awarded partial costs to the GOC.

Action has been taken against an individual for supplying spectacles to a minor when not appearing in any of the relevant registers. At a Magistrates Court the individual was found guilty on two counts and fined £250 for each offence.

More recently, considerable discussion has been raised by the GOC action against a company supplying contact lenses direct to the public. The situation was determined by what constituted supervision of such sales. A Magistrates Court found in favour of the GOC and the two individuals concerned were ordered to pay a total of £50,000 prosecution costs and fines totalling £500 each (the level of fine taking into account the size of the costs awarded against the defendants).

Handing Over Prescriptions

A number of practitioners have been found guilty of failure to comply with the Act by not providing a copy of the patient's prescription at the end of the examination. A recent case was brought against a locum domiciliary optometrist for failing to supply eight patients at a retirement home with the necessary prescription. The GOC acted on the basis that failure to hand over the prescription constituted serious professional misconduct. The practitioner was found guilty and fined £250. At the hearing of a similar case in 1995 the individual was found guilty of failure to hand over the prescription in addition to other charges and was fined £750.

Charging before Testing a Patient

The GOC heard a case in 1995, one of the elements of which was asking the patient to pay a fee prior to an examination being carried out. In this instance it was found that the optometrist involved was not responsible for the demand for payment and that it was a practice issue. The view was taken however that the Opticians Act is very specific in providing that a person should not be required to pay a fee in advance of the test.

Conviction for a Criminal Offence

Many of the cases considered by the GOC relate to individuals who have been found guilty of criminal offences. The spread of these cases is wide ranging from sexual offences to causing death by dangerous driving and from fraud to misleading advertising. The route is there for the GOC to follow up on *any* conviction in a court for a criminal offence.

The above has looked carefully at the Opticians Act and the legal bases established by the Act. A very important element however that has not been discussed in detail was the establishment of the GOC. There are further areas of professional requirements that are established by subordinate rulings from the GOC and the constitution, powers and rules established by the GOC will be reviewed in Chapter 8.

Key points 1: General aspects of the Opticians Act

1 The GOC was established
2 Regulations to allow the GOC to make subordinate legislation were provided
3 Registers of optometrists, dispensing opticians, bodies corporate were established
4 Standards for education and training were set

Key points 2: Criminal offences affecting non-registered 'opticians'

1 Pretending to have the required qualifications to enable registration with the GOC
2 Pretending to appear in any of the registers maintained by the GOC when not qualified to so appear
3 Use of any of the titles protected under the Act
4 Supply of spectacles or contact lenses (other than 'ready readers') without a valid written prescription
5 Fitting of contact lenses when not having an appropriate qualification
6 Testing eyes when not appearing in the relevant register

Key points 3: Offences by individuals registered with the GOC

1 Conviction for a criminal offence
2 Charging a fee before providing an examination
3 Failing to carry out an examination with due care and attention
4 Failing to hand over a prescription at the end of an examination
5 Failing to issue a written statement as required at the end of an examination
6 Failing to comply with GOC regulations

8

The General Optical Council

As described in Chapter 7, the main consequence of the Opticians Act 1958 was the establishment of the General Optical Council (GOC) and the subsequent registration of optometrists and dispensing opticians. Both the Opticians Act 1958 and the Opticians Act 1989 require the GOC to establish a number of committees.

Committees

Education Committee

The Education Committee was established under the terms of the Opticians Act 1958 as an advisory committee to the GOC on all matters relating to optical training and examinations. The main functions were seen as advising the Council on the promotion of high standards of professional education of optometrists and dispensing opticians and also on the supervision of training institutions and the qualifying examinations.

The Opticians Act required that, in addition to the GOC members, the committee included one person representing those persons training student optometrists, one person representing those persons training student dispensing opticians, and one person nominated by the Minister of Education. In order to fulfil its role regarding the promotion of high standards in supervision of training institutions and qualifying examinations, the council appoints a panel of 16 persons, from various disciplines, from whom 'visitors' are drawn. It is the function of members of the panel to visit and report on standards, when requested.

Amending rules were made as SI 1974/149, SI 1984/1249 and most recently as SI 1999/1211. The result of these amendments is that the current composition of the Education Committee is:

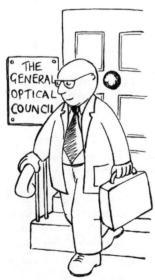

1 Three members of the council from among the persons nominated by the Privy Council one of whom shall be the person nominated by the Privy Council as specially qualified to advise the council on educational problems generally.
2 Two members of the council representing registered optometrists.
3 Three members of the council representing registered dispensing opticians.
4 The members of the council nominated by the College of Optometrists (2).
5 The nominated member of the council representing those engaged in the education or examination of persons training as optometrists.
6 Two members of the council from among the persons nominated by the Royal College of Ophthalmologists.
7 With effect from 1 January 2002 the member of the council nominated by the Association of Dispensing Opticians.

In addition the council shall appoint to the committee from outside the council:

1 One person appearing to the council to represent persons training student optometrists.
2 One person appearing to the council to represent persons training student dispensing opticians.
3 One person nominated by the Secretary of State.

All appointments to the committee shall be for a period of 1 year expiring on 31 December. The functions of the committee remain unchanged.

The Companies Committee

The role of this committee was again advisory offering information on all matters (other than disciplinary) relating to bodies corporate carrying on business as ophthalmic or dispensing opticians. In addition to the council members, the act required that the committee membership should include at least one person representing the interests of bodies corporate carrying on business as ophthalmic opticians and at least one person representing the interests of bodies corporate carrying on business as dispensing opticians.

The composition of the committee was revised by SI 1994/2579 and currently consists of:

1 Four members of council including at least one member:
   (a) nominated by the Privy Council
   (b) chosen to represent the interests of registered optometrists
   (c) chosen to represent the interests of dispensing opticians.
2 Four persons not on the council who appear to the council to represent the interests of bodies corporate carrying on business as ophthalmic opticians.
3 Three persons not on the council who appear to the council to represent the interests of bodies corporate carrying on business as dispensing opticians.
4 A registered medical practitioner who represents the interests of registered medical practitioners engaged in the testing of sight in the practices of bodies corporate and who may or may not be a council member.

All appointments are made for a period of 1 year expiring on 31 December.

Additional committees

Section 19 of the act makes provision for the GOC to establish additional committees for any purpose other than a purpose expressly required by the act. The council has the authority to set the number of members in any such additional committee, and also the term of office of members. Any such committee can include members who are not GOC members, providing that at least two-thirds of the members of any such committee are council members. At present committees set up under this section are:

1 Miscellaneous Affairs Committee
2 Professional Conduct Committee
3 Finance and Procedure Committee
4 Contact Lens Committee.

The GOC Role in Training

The power of the council extends from granting, where appropriate, the status of 'approved training institution' for new training providers to reviewing regularly the status of existing already approved institutions. It also provides for approval of a qualification as an 'approved qualification' if it appears appropriate.

The term training covers the period of study at an 'approved training institution' and the pre-registration period up to successful completion of the pre-qualifying examinations (PQEs). This means that in addition to the training institutions of:

- Anglia Polytechnic University
- University of Aston in Birmingham
- Bradford University
- The City University in London
- Glasgow Caledonian University
- University of Manchester Institute of Science and Technology
- University of Ulster
- University of Wales College, Cardiff.

The GOC also has responsibility for ensuring the examinations carried out by the College of Optometrists are to the required standard and that pre-registration supervision is adequate.

To comply with the terms of the Opticians Act defining those entitled to test sight the Council has made regulations for exemption to accommodate those training to become optometrists and other relevant groups. These can be found in SI 1994/70 and subsequent amendment SI 1999/2897.

The GOC has also recently looked at the area of continuing education and training (CET) for optometrists and is currently looking to introduce a requirement for registered optometrists to complete a minimum amount of CET. The proposal is for 30 hours of CET to be completed over a 3-year period. It is likely that the College of Optometry and ABDO accreditation process for CET will be used to determine whether or not training is provided at an acceptable standard.

Rules made by the GOC

Rules on referral

The Opticians Act 1958 made special reference to the need for rules to be formulated relating to disease or injury to the eye. This duty has been carried forward into Section 31(5) of the Opticians Act 1989, which states:

> The Council shall make and submit to the Privy Council rules providing that where it appears to a registered optician that a person consulting him is suffer-

ing from an injury or disease of the eye, the optician shall, except in an emergency or where that person is consulting him for the purpose of being given treatment under rules 'relating to orthoptics' or in such other cases as may be prescribed, being cases in which it is, owing to special circumstances, impracticable or inexpedient to do so, take the prescribed steps to refer that person to a registered medical practitioner for advice and treatment.

The original GOC rules were embodied in SI 1960/1936 and remained unchanged until the 1999 revision (SI 1999/3267 The General Optical Council (Rules relating to Injury or Disease of the Eye) Order of Council 1999). The latest rules have incorporated a number of minor amendments that will have a profound effect on Optometry. The main disadvantage of the original rules was that as practice and clinical skills moved forward optometrists were better able to identify abnormalities and monitor minor conditions rather than refer but in so doing they were effectively breaking the rules. If on the other hand they were to refer every patient that was seen who presented with an abnormality the Hospital Eye Service (HES) would be unable to cope. The result was that most practitioners with the tacit approval of other eye care specialists 'bent' the rules. The latest modifications take account of the situation that had developed.

The rules state:

1 If a patient attending a registered optician appears to be suffering from an injury or disease of the eye, of which the patient's general medical practitioner may be unaware, then a report of any findings must be sent to the general practitioner (GP).
2 When referring, the following procedure should be followed:
   (a) Advise the patient to consult their medical practitioner.
   (b) Wherever possible, send to the registered medical practitioner named by the patient a written report of findings indicating the grounds for thinking that injury or disease of the eye is present.
   (c) If action appears urgent, then such measures as are available to inform the general medical practitioner immediately, for example, telephone, shall be taken.
3 If a patient is unwilling to consult their GP despite the advice of a registered optician on conscientious or any other grounds then this must be recorded and the details given. (To protect against potential litigation, although not in the Rules, the professional body has advised practitioners that the patient should sign and date the record indicating agreement with the content.)
4 If in the professional judgement of an optometrist or dispensing optician there is no justification to refer or referral would be impracticable or inexpedient the optometrist may decide not to refer but should
   (a) record a description of the injury or disease noted
   (b) give reasons for not referring
   (c) record details of any advice given to patients and if appropriate and with the consent of the patient notify the GP of the action and reasons.
5 A dispensing optician may decide to refer a patient to an optometrist in which case the same details should be recorded as are outlined in 4 above.
6 None of the regulations regarding referral shall prevent an optician from rendering in an emergency whatever services are in the best interests of the person consulting him or her or carrying out orthoptic treatment if considered appropriate.

These rules by the GOC place a greater duty on the registered optician to refer a patient than do the National Health Service (NHS) Terms of Service which simply require the GP to be informed.

The rules laid down in SI 1989/1176 The Sight Testing (Examination and Prescription) Regulations 1989 also affect disease and injury and complement the GOC rules. They are made under the Terms of Section 26(1) of the Opticians Act 1989 and are incorporated as an amendment to the Opticians Act 1958 imposed by the Health and Medicines Act 1988. The requirement in Section 3(1)(a) of SI 1989/1176 is that it shall be the duty of a doctor or optometrist testing the sight of another person to perform for the purpose of detecting signs of injury, disease or abnormality in the eye or elsewhere:

1 An examination of the external surface of the eye and its immediate vicinity.
2 An intra-ocular examination, either by means of an ophthalmoscope or by such other means as the doctor or optometrist considers appropriate.
3 Such additional examinations as appear clinically necessary.

Rules on publicity

The GOC made its first rules on publicity in 1964 and these have been the source of much debate in subsequent years, particularly following the Office of Fair Trading Report (1982) and the efforts of Lord Rugby to introduce 'ready readers' into the optical market. The suggestions were for relaxation of the publicity rules to allow wider freedom to advertise and thereby, in theory, increase competition. Further pressure was placed on the GOC with the introduction of the Health and Social Security Act 1984, which allowed a wider marketing of spectacles and opened up competition to both registered and unqualified suppliers.

At this time the GOC submitted rules to the Privy Council but these were not found acceptable to the Privy Council on the grounds that the proposed Rules were still too restrictive. In normal circumstances the rules would have been returned to the GOC for further modification but using the powers granted under the new Health and Social Security Act 1984 the Privy Council drew up and imposed their own set of regulations which were then, after formal agreement by the GOC, issued as SI 1985/203.

Under the terms of these rules, which are still in force at present, a registered optician or an enrolled body corporate may use publicity in relation to practice or business providing that:

1 It is legal, decent, honest and truthful.
2 It does not bring the profession into disrepute.
3 It does not contain any reference to the efficiency of facilities provided by other registered opticians or bodies corporate.
4 Any claims made are capable of substantiation.
5 No claims are made suggesting superiority over any other practice or business.

The changes in regulations prompted a dramatic increase in the number of registered practitioners prepared to advertise. The type, style and quality of advertisements are inevitably variable and it has to be said that many advertisements came extremely close to breaking the regulations. Taste is obviously a very personal factor and it seems that experience is helping to improve the quality of advertising albeit slowly. The wider use of advertising agencies with an open brief has in the past led to some registered opticians falling foul of the rules.

Rules on contact lenses

Before June 1985, the GOC had not published rules on the fitting and supply of contact lenses. The council had, however, issued guidance on these matters which had been regularly updated and which before the introduction of rules in 1985 came within the simple statement:

> In order to protect both individual patients and the public at large, it must be made clear that in relation to all registered opticians' professional activities, it is beholden upon the individual to maintain the highest standards of experience, training, performance and behaviour.

Many practitioners felt that this was inadequate and the GOC itself drew up draft regulations for contact lens practice which were rejected by the Privy Council on the grounds that the proposed rules were outside the scope of the legal duty of the GOC.

Under the terms of the Opticians Act 1958, the GOC was given permission to make rules prohibiting or regulating the prescription, supply and fitting of contact lenses by registered opticians, enrolled bodies corporate, and their employees, but not covering subsequent follow-up of the patient.

The Health and Social Security Act 1984 introduced a new section to the Opticians Act 1958, to deal with certain aspects of contact lens work. Section 25 of the Opticians Act 1989, the new section restricts the fitting of contact lenses to:

1 registered opticians
2 registered medical practitioners
3 recognized medical students.

In addition, the GOC was required to make regulations covering the fitting of contact lenses by training opticians and to submit these for approval to the Privy Council. The final sub-section dealt with the punishment for contravening these regulations.

It was, therefore, in June 1985 that SI 1985/886 was published as 'The General Optical Council (Rules on the Fitting of Contact Lenses) Order of Council 1985'. The rules specified those groups of opticians in addition to those already qualified who may fit contact lenses as:

1 opticians engaged in approved basic training
2 pre-registration students
3 holders of partially recognized overseas qualifications who have concluded supplementary training in the UK
4 those engaged in training for a higher contact lens qualification.

The rules also required that for any groups outlined above, contact lenses could only be fitted if under the continuous personal supervision of a registered optician or registered medical practitioner.

The Contact Lens (Qualifications, etc.) Rules 1988 were issued by the GOC, coming into force on 1 September 1988. SI 1988/1305. Under the terms of the new regulations, a registered optician is not allowed to fit a contact lens without either:

1 an approved qualification
2 certification
3 provisional certification or
4 adequate supervision.

A list of approved qualifications is published in Appendix A of the new rules as amended by SI 1989/375 and reproduced in Table 8.1. The regulations

Table 8.1   Approved qualifications for fitting of contact lenses

Short description appearing in register

Qualification A
Any qualification recognized as entitling the holder to be first registered as an ophthalmic optician after 31 December 1960

Qualification B
Any of the following additional qualifications:
The Fellowship of the British College of Ophthalmic Opticians (Optometrists) including the Contact Lens Module FBCO (subsequently MCOptom)

The Diploma in Contact Lens Practice of the British Optical Association DCLP

The Contact Lens Certificate of the Scottish Association of Opticians DCLP

The Supplementary Contact Lens Certificate of the Worshipful Company of Spectacle Makers cLcert.(SMc)

The Supplementary Contact Lens Diploma of the British Optical Association cLCert.(BOA)

The Diploma in Contact Lens Practice of the British College of Ophthalmic Opticians (Optometrists) DCLP

The Contact Lens Diploma of the Association of Dispensing Opticians:
    For persons who are Fellows of the Association FADO (Hons) lcL
    For other persons CL (ADO)

The Contact Lens Diploma of the Association of British Dispensing Opticians:
    For persons who are Fellows of the Association FBDO (Hons) CL
    For other persons t2L (ABDO)

The Diploma in Contact Lens Fitting of the Faculty of Dispensing Opticians DCLF

The Contact Lens Certificate of the Association of British Dispensing Opticians FBDO (CLI)

Contact Lens Practice (Supplementary) Qualification of the British College of Optometrists:
    For persons who are Members of the College MBCO
    For persons who are Fellows of the College FBCO

mean that any newly qualified optometrist is entitled to fit lenses by virtue of having passed the contact lens examination section of the PQEs. Dispensing opticians, on the other hand, are in the future required to take a supplementary examination to achieve an approved qualification. The regulations also remove the right of optometrists who qualified before 1960 to fit contact lenses without obtaining certification. The date is chosen as the first date at which contact lenses were examined for qualification as a registered optometrist. The date appeared earlier in Notice N1O of the GOC in relation to annotation in the register.

To obtain certification an applicant had to show:

1 Evidence of holding an approved qualification.
2 Evidence of having fitted a minimum of 150 patients in the previous 3 years.
3 Current involvement in teaching contact lens practice and evidence of involvement for at least 3 years in the full-time instruction of persons training as opticians in an approved training institution.

It was possible to obtain professional certification if:

1 a registered optician anticipated that he would have fitted contact lenses to at least 150 persons in the period from September 1986 to September 1989
2 undertaking, or about to undertake, a course of study leading, after examination, to an approved qualification.

The final cut-off date for those not meeting the new requirements was 31 December 1990. This move prompted considerable anger from practitioners who qualified before 1960, the argument against the rules being that they remove an existing right that such practitioners have to fit lenses. The GOC has tried to make certification relatively straightforward.

The British College of Optometrists (BCO) obtained GOC approval to set a supplementary examination in contact lenses for optometrists falling outside the scope of SI 1988/1305.

A further GOC ruling relating to contact lenses has been introduced and that is the Contact Lens Specification Rules 1989. According to these rules it shall be the duty of an optician to give a person whom he/she has fitted with a contact lens a written prescription immediately following the final fitting. The information provided must be adequate to allow replication of the lens by another person. The exception would be that an optician would not be required to supply information to an optician who is not qualified to fit contact lenses under the provision of SI 1988/1305.

The advent of internet services has meant that patients are able to purchase lenses from non-clinical sources provided to the specification that a clinician has to provide. Often these lenses are considerably cheaper but include no provision for after-care of the patient. The GOC still believes it is the duty of a practitioner to ensure the continuing clinical well being of the patient but this is obviously extremely difficult if the patient can purchase lenses and solutions elsewhere. The practitioner has a duty to inform a patient of due after-care but if the patient fails to attend what is the position? It would be considered normal to attempt recall more than once but if there is no response the practitioner is advised to contact the patient in writing indicating that without after-care no responsibility can be taken for any damage that occurs to the eyes. New GOC rules have been proposed which would separate out the clinical care and the product provision allowing provision by non-qualified suppliers. Under the terms of the proposed regulations due to be enacted in 2001 a specification would be valid for a specified period but this period would not need to coincide with the period recommended for after-care. The practitioner would only be responsible for the clinical care of a patient for a 6-month period from the date of initial fitting unless the patient continued to attend the practice at regular intervals specified by the practitioner.

The autumn of 1999 saw a further problem for contact lens practitioners. For some time it had been shown that there is a small risk of variant Creutzfeldt–Jacob disease being transmitted via corneal transplant. In late 1999 the government advisory committee on the disease (SEAC) decided that there was also a risk of transmission via contact lenses. There have been no reported cases and no contaminated contact lenses had been found but in response to the report the Medical Devices Agency introduced advice preventing the re-use of trial contact lenses. It has also warned against the use of contact devices for measuring intra-ocular pressure. The situation is unresolved and it would be expected that optometrists would take great care in the use of trial lenses and contact equipment until a final decision is made. The GOC has advised that the re-use of trial contact lenses introduces a risk of infection and should therefore be abandoned.

Rules on the sale of optical appliances

Following on from the Health and Social Security Act 1984, the GOC produced the Sale of Optical Appliances Order of Council 1984 SI 1984/1778 which came into effect in December 1984. This order deals with sale of appliances by non-qualified persons to anyone other than:

1 a person under 16 years of age
2 a person registered blind or partially sighted.

It covers the normal range of complete spectacles, frames and lenses but still does not permit the sale of contact lenses or low vision aids by the unregistered. For the person under 16, no appliance can be supplied by a person not registered and for the registered blind and partially sighted anything other than empty frames can only be supplied by a registered practitioner. In order to protect the general public SI 1984/1778 lays down certain conditions that must be fulfilled for the sale to be considered as falling within the terms of the Health and Social Security Act 1984. These conditions fall into three basic headings:

1 Safety and serviceability conditions:
   (a) no appliance can be supplied which contains any cellulose nitrate or celluloid
   (b) all lenses supplied must conform to the requirements of Appendix A of BS 2738: Part 1: 1989 dealing with surface defects and quality of glazing

(c) all lenses supplied of glass or plastic material must conform to the requirements of BS 3062: 1985.

2 Optical performance conditions: In this section, the conditions are in two parts and relate either to non-complex spectacles which are defined as:

(a) spectacles prescribed for reading only

(b) spectacles with single vision spherical lenses and having a positive power not exceeding 5.00 dioptres.

Spectacles not falling within the above two categories are considered as complex.

The conditions relating to all spectacles whether they are complex or not are:

(a) The spectacles must be made according to a written prescription produced by the customer which:
   (i) has been provided by a registered medical practitioner or registered optometrist following a sight test
   (ii) is dated not more than 2 years prior to presentation.

(b) The completed spectacles must conform to the requirements of BS 2738: Part 1: 1989 and be within the tolerances set out in Clauses 6–12 of BS 2738: 1962 to be considered as in accordance with the written prescription.

Those additional conditions relating to complex spectacles are as follows:

(a) the spectacles must be verified by focimeter as matching the written prescription

(b) the spectacles must have their lenses centred according to the customer's interpupillary distance (unless otherwise specified)

(c) if a back vertex distance is specified on the written prescription, then the retailer or staff must check the back vertex distance and make any allowances that may be required to produce the necessary optical effect.

3 Customer redress conditions: In order to safeguard the customer's rights in the event of the spectacles being unsatisfactory the following conditions apply:

(a) the conditions relating to safety and serviceability and to optical performance form part of the retailer's contract with the customer

(b) the retailer cannot contract to take away or vary the customer's rights in relation to Section 14 of the Sale of Goods Act 1979, or Section 13 of the Supply of Goods and Services Act 1982.

Overseas Qualifications

The GOC have agreed that with the exception of the Fellowship Diploma of the Association of Ophthalmic Opticians, Ireland no overseas qualification has been found to be similar in subject matter and standard to the UK qualification and therefore to receive recognition.

However, many overseas qualifications do offer a standard and content adequate enough to be considered for partial recognition. If, therefore, a person comes to the UK as the holder of a qualification given partial recognition they will be expected to succeed at examinations as prescribed by the GOC before being granted permission to register to practise in the UK.

Normally the examinations shall include a general oral including legal aspects of practice and a practical examination covering a routine eye examination together with such additional papers as deemed necessary.

General Guidelines

In the past the GOC have regularly produced booklets to complement the general rules and regulations relating to optometry. These booklets contained guidance on interpretation of the rules.

Following the publication of Notice N22 in March 1987 (the updated Notice for the Guidance of the Profession) the GOC decided to withdraw all guidance and to rely on the rules alone. If there were any need for interpretation then this would be left to individuals. It was decided however that where the matter related to general conduct then the Guidance of peer groups such as the BCO may be taken as an indication of the professional feeling on particular matters.

The College of Optometrists' guidelines are discussed in Chapter 13.

Key points 1: The GOC may make rules relating to the following areas

1 The use of publicity
2 The use of business names
3 The administration of drugs in the course of practice
4 The practice of orthoptics
5 The sale of optical appliances
6 The prescribing, fitting and supply of contact lenses in the course of practice
7 Injury or disease of the eye

Key points 2: GOC committees

1 Education
2 Companies
3 Miscellaneous affairs
4 Standards
5 Finance & procedure
6 Investigating
7 Disciplinary

Key points 3: Membership of the GOC as of January 2001

1 Eight persons nominated by the Privy Council, one of whom will be Chair
2 Six persons elected by registered optometrists
3 Five persons elected to represent dispensing opticians
4 Four persons appointed by the Royal College of Ophthalmologists
5 Two members appointed by the College of Optometrists as examining body
6 Two members appointed by ABDO as examining body
7 One member appointed by the optometric training institutions

---

9

The Optical Services Audit Committee and the General Optical Council

The optometric profession throughout the 1980s came under tremendous pressure from legislative change. The Office of Fair Trading Report of 1982 seemed to release all the pressures that had been building since the Opticians Act 1958 received parliamentary approval. Chapter 7 on the Opticians Act 1989 catalogues the changes that resulted in legislation but does not discuss additional pressures that arose towards the end of the 1980s.

In the build up to the introduction of the Health and Medicines Act 1988, the government reviewed methods of producing efficiency in the optometric services and proposed for discussion the possibility of a so-called 'two-tier' service. To some groups, the idea of a quick, inexpensive check of the refractive error with no other requirements was extremely appealing. Others concerned with the overall health care of the population found the idea an affront to the professional services that had been available for many years and that had proved so valuable to patients in health screening for both ocular and general conditions. The argument hinged on the patients' ability to decide on which 'tier' would suit their specific needs, i.e. health check or just spectacle check.

The General Optical Council (GOC) took the initiative. By combining the issue of the 'two-tier' system with that of problems with unregistered sellers of spectacles and the introduction of new terms of service the GOC proposed to the Secretary of State for Health that it should undertake a review of optical services in the UK. Upon receiving approval for the proposal the GOC agreed on 3 July 1989, to appoint a committee to be called the Optical Service Audit Committee (OSAC). This was composed of the lay members of the GOC who could be seen to have no professional or commercial conflict of interest in the services. The terms of reference given by the GOC to the committee were:

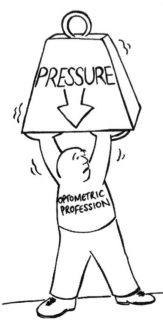

> To consider how the present and future needs of the public for the care of its vision and for the health of its eyes can best be met, by whom, and with what training and qualifications; and with what built in protection for the public, in accordance with the General Optical Council's general duty to protect the public.

The OSAC was to take information from the professional bodies concerned and all other organizations and individuals having an interest in the services and willing to take part. To assist the committee, three specialist advisers were appointed covering the disciplines of ophthalmology, optometry and dispensing optics.

Consultation was wide and evidence was accumulated from many different sources. In addition to meeting specific groups with a known interest and background in eye care the committee held a public open meeting on the eye care services. Groups and individuals were invited to respond to specific questions that arose during the course of the review and the committee arranged to see various aspects of eye care services for itself. Eventually, 1 year after starting its work, the OSAC produced its report. The report had great impact on the eye care services and will be discussed as the implementation process still continues today.

In the introduction the OSAC indicates that it took the objectives of the review to be as follows: 'To propose, on the basis of evidence received, a framework for optical services in the UK from 1990 onwards: and to identify those areas in which modification or development of the existing structure would be desirable for the public benefit, both in vision care and value for money in its delivery.'

The review took place against a background of legislative change, including deregulation of much of optical dispensing, including the introduction of the sale of over-the-counter reading spectacles and the abolition of the right to a National Health Service (NHS) sight test for an estimated 60% of the population.

The report itself is divided into eight review and discussion chapters and two summary chapters. There are, in addition, a number of appendices giving background and detailed information for readers. The sections may for convenience be taken in terms of professional eye care, the organization and future developments of optical services, consumer interests and the European Community (EC) effect.

Professional Eye Care

The report briefly outlines the relative roles of those responsible for eye care in the UK who are given as ophthalmologists, ophthalmic medical practitioners, general medical practitioners, optometrists, dispensing opticians and orthoptists, and follows this by reviewing the content of the sight test. A sight test has been taken as meaning 'a refraction and a full eye examination and such additional examinations which may be considered as clinically necessary for the patient', as laid down in the Sight Testing (Examination and Prescription) Regulations SI 1989/1176. This definition is in agreement with the objectives of the 'sight test' as defined by the British College of Optometrists (BCO) in its guidance:

1 to detect ocular abnormality
2 to specify functional corrections for defects of sight
3 to suggest or provide remedial visual training where appropriate.

The review by the OSAC investigated whether there was a need to maintain the above definition and objectives or whether the public's need could be met by alternative testing methods including a direct review of the 'two-tier' proposal. This area obviously proved extremely difficult due to the many diverse arguments for retention of the status quo and as many for removal of the existing legislation, to allow anyone to provide a rapid spectacle check.

The committee investigated self-selection of spectacles by patients, the use of auto-refractors and the possible provision by dispensing opticians of spectacle testing only. The report recommends however that the 'integrity of the sight test according to current statutory regulations should be maintained as a minimum standard in the present state of public knowledge of the sight test and eye care generally, and in the present state of visual care technology'.

In commenting on the two-tier proposal, the OSAC did note that if public awareness were to increase to a point where informed choice by patients was possible and there were technical advances with improved performance of equipment, then a 5-year reassessment may provide a different outcome. They also noted that it might be possible to train dispensing opticians to be capable of carrying out aspects of refraction under supervision by whoever completes the eye examination and prescribes. This latter situation has subsequently been established. In order for the objective of the OSAC to be achieved it is also recommended that both the professional bodies and the government should carefully monitor:

1 the incidence of eye disease and the numbers of sight tests performed, both analysed in age groups
2 public awareness of vision care
3 the impact of new technology on practice.

Direct Referral from Optometrists to Ophthalmologists

In reviewing the optical services, the report provides a number of recommendations relating to inter-professional activity. A major change to the existing procedures that the OSAC supported was the direct referral of patients to ophthalmologists when it was suspected that disease or disorder was present. To achieve this it noted that clear criteria needed to be agreed upon between the professions and a system of notification to the general medical practitioners established. This is also now happening through co-management schemes for dealing with cataract and glaucoma referrals.

Also recommended was the monitoring of the consequences of the abolition of the NHS sight test to large numbers of the population. There were suggestions that there would be either a resultant drop in early detection of ocular disease and subsequently an increase in workload of eye departments or, alternatively, a switch of patients wanting only eye examinations to ophthalmological departments thereby overloading the system. This would be particularly important with the anticipated demographic shifts in the 1990s towards an older patient population. Early reports showed that the number of pathologies detected in the first year of the new legislation were markedly reduced and following subsequent lobbying the NHS eye examination eligibility was reinstated for the over 60 year olds.

The committee recommended a reversal of the overloading trend for hospital clinics and suggested that ophthalmologists, medical practitioners and optometrists discuss together ways of delegating to optometrists routine ophthalmological tasks to attempt to relieve the overload in the eye department of some NHS hospitals. There was a recommendation that contractual arrangements should be made between hospitals, general medical practitioners and optometric practices and medical eye centres for the continued sight testing and monitoring of certain diseases in patients which would relieve hospital clinics of routine check-ups. It was concluded that the experience of the optometrist in the area of primary eye care would be a valuable way to relieve general medical practitioners of routine tasks relating to eye care for which they have little training. All of these are now in place to various degrees although there is still a long way to go in building trust before they are accepted as normal.

Equipment and Continuing Education

An area of concern to the OSAC was standard of equipment in practice. There is no specific list of equipment that should be available in a practice and indeed the College of Optometrists when considering this found it extremely difficult to produce such a list. The College has provided a breakdown of the basic eye examination requirements and indicated that suitable equipment was needed. In addition a list of equipment was available for pre-registration supervisors to ensure adequate training opportunities.

The level of equipment in practice has steadily improved in no small measure due to the influx of new corporate business. There are also now steps being taken to provide through clinical governance assessment of the competency of practitioners in the use of the equipment. This latter aspect also falls in line with the GOC moves to establish continuing education as a precondition to continued registration. This is of particular importance because of rapid advances in both clinical knowledge and technical optical advances.

Rationalization of Functions

A final development in organization foreseen by the OSAC was the rationalization of the optical bodies and in particular the College of Optometrists, the Association of Optometrists, the Association of British Dispensing Opticians (ABDO), the Institute of Optometry and the British Orthoptic Society. Many of the functions undertaken by the different bodies and the training needs of their members overlap and for efficiency and economy, and also for better public awareness, it was suggested there should be a rationalization of their functions. This has not proved easy as the individual bodies have been independent for a considerable time. There are now joint groups such as the inter-professional group where all of the main players are represented and meet at regular intervals.

Consumer Interests

The underlying theme of the OSAC report was public benefit and protection and it is not surprising therefore that most attention has been paid to this area. The need for better promotion of information about entitlement to the NHS sight test and also entitlement towards supply of spectacles following examination was expressed. It was suggested, there was a need to simplify the booklet and procedures that patients were required to complete if they wished to apply for assistance towards examination and spectacle supply.

Also it was suggested, there should be a major effort to inform particular groups such as parents of young children, drivers and the visually handicapped of the range of services available and the benefits of regular examination. It was proposed that the Department of Health and the Health Education Authority, together with professional bodies, should work to achieve this end.

Optometric Outlets

The downward trend in volume of patients attending for eye examination following removal of NHS eligibility and rapid expansion of some optical companies provoked concern for the future of smaller independent and rural practices. It was not considered in the public interest for these to disappear and the OSAC recommended that the GOC should monitor year by year:

1 the relative numbers of practices owned by corporate bodies and by independent practitioners
2 comparative share of the market of the different types of practice
3 comparative numbers of sight tests conducted in each.

This was in line with reservations put forward in the Crook report which formed the basic discussion document for the introduction of the 1958 Opticians Act (see Chapter 7).

Consumer Issues

With the specific interests of the consumer in mind the committee reviewed the areas of contact lenses, over-the-counter reading spectacles, pricing and prescription hand-over.

The results of their discussions and deliberations were contained in a series of recommendations. In contact lenses much had recently been achieved through the GOC contact lens registration qualification rules and it was suggested that this area should be further reviewed with the intention of providing the best possible consumer service and safety at competitive costs.

Since changes in legislation required optometrists either to hand a copy of the prescription to the patient immediately following the examination or a copy of a statement indicating that no spectacles were required there had been practitioners who took exception to the law. It was, however, considered to the patient's benefit to be able to 'shop' for appliances and the committee recommended that all practitioners should be reminded of their duty to hand-over the prescription.

On the other hand, the legislation allowing the purchase of ready-made reading spectacles was questioned on the basis of ability accurately to assess needs without examination. A recommendation was made that all sales of ready-made spectacles should be accompanied by a clearly worded recommendation that the purchaser should have a sight test.

Changes in legislation removing the NHS rights to examination and spectacles removed the previous complaint procedure that was within the control of the NHS Family Practitioner Committees. This meant that many patients were unable to follow any form of independent complaint procedure that was obviously an unsatisfactory situation. A complaint procedure already existed within the profession via the Association of Optometrists who pass any complaint to the relevant organization or individual for the most effective action but this was not seen as independent.

The report recommended that the GOC and the professional bodies should review the situation and propose a formal complaints procedure that would be independent, easily accessible, rapid and able to provide binding arbitration. The method of financing of such a scheme was recognized as requiring careful consideration, particularly if the proposal to appoint an independent ombudsman was accepted. This has now progressed and the Optical Consumer Complaint Service has been established (see Chapter 6).

European Community

The EC Directive on the recognition of higher education diplomas to allow the movement of professionals throughout Europe was carefully considered. In its view, although OSAC offered no recommendations the timescale for any development was very long and it was expected that optometrists in the continent would seek to achieve the UK standard and to this end the GOC would control certification and monitor UK standards.

The Future

This report carefully studied evidence from all sectors involved with eye care, including the consumer. After weighing up all the evidence presented, the OSAC provided a series of opinions and recommendations together with a list of areas that required further consideration. While there were some sectors of the eye care service that felt disappointed at the minimal progress provided to their own aspirations, the report as a whole seemed to have produced well balanced conclusions many of which have now been initiated.

This report provided the basic groundwork from which each professional group could progress, albeit perhaps at different rates than proposed. The proposals and recommendations placed responsibility firmly on the shoulders of all those professions working within the eye care field to produce mutually agreeable reforms for the benefit of the patient and for the more efficient use of their respective times.

As a blueprint for the future it provided a basic framework while providing enough manoeuvrability for individual groups to finalize the overall design. Activity through OSAC at the GOC is still ongoing and still helping to drive forward new concepts on eye care provision.

The National Health Service (NHS) regulations regarding ophthalmic practice and the general investigation procedures have been dealt with in Chapters 5 and 6. There is a further disciplinary process, however, which is governed by the General Optical Council (GOC). Although the two may well interact, they have different outcomes. The NHS procedures relate to a contractor having broken the terms of service for practitioners as laid down in the relevant statutory instruments; the GOC procedures are much more far reaching and can relate to anything which may pertain to the practitioner in an ophthalmic practice situation. The outcome of the two procedures is also different in that the NHS investigation may result in prohibition to practise within the health service while the GOC investigation may result in erasure of the practitioner's name from the lists and total prohibition to practise.

Scope of GOC Discipline

As laid down in Sections 14–23 of the Opticians Act 1989 and regulated by SI 1960/1934, SI 1960/1935, SI 1961/1239 and SI 1961/1933, the GOC has the right to investigate any breach of professional discipline. In this connection there are two committees, established under the Opticians Act 1958, and maintained by the Opticians Act 1989: the Investigation Committee carries out the preliminary investigation, and the Disciplinary Committee considers and decides sufficiently serious disciplinary cases referred to them by the Investigating Committee. In the case of a decision by the Disciplinary Committee to strike the name of a registered optician from the register, there exists the right of appeal against the decision, to the Judicial Committee of the Privy Council.

The disciplinary jurisdiction covers the following offences:

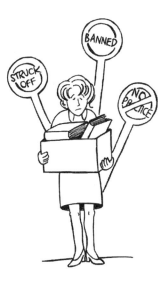

1 A criminal offence, other than a trivial one, by a registered optician.
2 Infamous conduct in any professional respect by a registered optician.
3 Any offence by a body corporate under the terms of the Opticians Act 1989.
4 Failure by a body corporate to observe the required conditions of enrolment.
5 Connivance by a body corporate at conduct leading to the erasure from the register of the name of a registered optician in its employ.
6 Breach of the rules made under Section 31 of the Opticians Act 1989 relating to
  (a) publicity
  (b) the name under which business is carried out

(c) the administering of drugs

(d) the prescription, supply and fitting of contact lenses.

7 Failure to make adequate arrangements for the fitting and supply of optical appliances.

8 Entries in a register or list made on fraudulent or incorrect grounds.

Composition of the Investigating Committee

The Investigating Committee has no special procedure laid down and ordinary committee procedure applies. At present the Chairman of the GOC may not be a member of this committee. The committee is made up of six members of council, two of whom are lay members, one an ophthalmologist, two representatives of ophthalmic opticians and one representative of dispensing opticians. If the dispensing representative declares an interest in a particular case then his place is taken by either an ophthalmologist or a lay member of the council. If the case is to be against a body corporate then the committee may co-opt either an ophthalmic representative or a dispensing representative of corporate bodies, depending upon the allegation.

Procedure for the Investigating Committee

A brief outline of the general procedure is as follows.

The Registrar of the GOC receives a complaint that a registered optician has committed a disciplinary offence. The complainant is required to supply one or more statutory declarations concerning the offence. The whole matter is then referred to the Chairman of the Investigating Committee, who decides whether to refer the matter to the Investigating Committee or to deal with the matter in some alternative way. In the case of a committee meeting being called, documentary evidence only is considered; there is no formal examination of witnesses or oral evidence. Although all parties are entitled to submit observations, no one is entitled to be present during the committee's deliberations. It is the function of the committee, when so called upon, to decide whether the case is sufficiently serious to be referred to the Disciplinary Committee.

Composition of the Disciplinary Committee

The committee as laid down in SI 1998/1338 is to consist of 15 members of the council appointed by the council made up as follows:

1 Three members from among those appointed by the Privy Council one of which will be chairman of the committee.

2 Two members from among the registered medical practitioners on council.

3 Four members from among those chosen to represent registered optometrists on council.

4 Three members from among those chosen to represent dispensing opticians on council.

5 Three further members from among those in the above categories not already selected.

The quorum for a committee is five and shall include a member of the committee appointed under each of 2, 3 and 4 above. If members are unable to be present due to a specific conflict of interest a member of council may be co-opted to the committee to provide a quorum.

Should the chairman of the committee be absent when a disciplinary case is due for hearing the committee shall elect one of its members present to preside as acting chairman.

The committee is required to meet at least once a year and all meetings would normally take place at the GOC offices in London although this is to change in 2001 when the offices of another professional body with better facilities will be used.

No person who has been on the Investigating Committee for a particular case may also sit on the Disciplinary Committee for that case.

Procedure for the Disciplinary Committee

The procedure for the Disciplinary Committee is set out in the General Optical Council (Disciplinary Committee) (Procedure) Order of Council 1985, SI 1985/1580. The preliminary proceedings are as follows:

1 A solicitor acting on behalf of the GOC, as soon as possible after referral of a disciplinary case to the committee, serves the respondent with a notice of enquiry, sent by registered mail or by recorded delivery. This notice should state the charge or charges and specify the alleged convictions or other facts relating to each charge, together with the day, time and place of the committee enquiry and should, in addition, contain a copy of the Opticians Act 1989 and a copy of SI 1985/1580.
2 If there is a complainant then the solicitor should also send him/her a copy of the notice of enquiry and SI 1985/1580.
3 An enquiry will not be held if a notice of enquiry has not been served in accordance with the above regulations.
4 An enquiry is not to be held within 28 days after the posting of the notice of enquiry, except with the agreement of the respondent.
5 The chairman may, if he/she so wishes, or upon application of any party to the investigation, postpone the hearing. The chairman may also refer a case to the Investigating Committee for further consideration as to whether an enquiry should be held. If any member of the committee feels that there is a need to amend the notice of enquiry then, if necessary, an amended notice should be sent to the respondent and the enquiry postponed.
6 The solicitor to the GOC should notify, as soon as possible, all the parties concerned if the enquiry is to be postponed.
7 Upon application by any party to the enquiry, the solicitor to the GOC sends to that party a copy of any relevant document received by the council from any party to the enquiry.

SI 1998/1337 allows for the interchange of information prior to a disciplinary hearing in an attempt to expedite the matter and provides that information should be served with regard to

- estimate of likely length of hearing
- a statement of the issues in the case
- how many witnesses are to be called
- what if any matters may be agreed without the need to call evidence
- any points of law which are expected to arise at the hearing.

The next stage after the preliminary proceedings is the hearing itself and the procedure for this is as follows:

1 The charge or charges are read in the presence of the respondent and of the complainant, if one appears. If the respondent does not attend, however, the committee may still continue and the charges are read out as if the respondent were present.
2 As soon as the charge or charges have been read out then the respondent, or his appointed agent, may object to all or part of the charge or charges made in point of law. Any other party may reply to any such objection. If the objection is upheld then no further proceedings will be taken on the section or sections to which the objection was raised.
3 The chairman asks the respondent at this stage whether all or any of the alleged facts or convictions in the charge or charges are submitted.
4 The complainant or his agent or the solicitor to the GOC then opens the case and may call witnesses and adduce evidence of any facts not admitted by the respondent which may be relevant. The respondent, or his appointed agent, may cross-examine any witness brought forward and the witness thereafter may be re-examined.
5 The respondent may then either:
   (a) submit that the evidence called at the hearing does not establish the charge alleged or does not merit erasure of the name from the register and the committee may then consider any such submission; or
   (b) if no submission is made, or if the submission is not upheld by the committee, then the respondent or his agent may call witnesses and adduce evidence. Any such witness may be cross-examined by the complainant, his agent or the solicitor to the GOC and re-examined. The complainant, or his agent or the solicitor to the GOC may address the committee on any point of the law that the respondent or his agent may raise during his address following the examination of witnesses.
6 The committee now deliberate and are asked to decide, in relation to each charge which remains outstanding, whether the facts substantiate the charge.
7 In the case of the committee finding a charge proved, then the complainant, or his agent or the solicitor to the GOC, is required to adduce evidence as to the circumstances leading up to the charge.
8 The respondent may then address the committee in mitigation and present any relevant evidence.
9 The committee are now required to decide whether they can properly reach a decision to make no disciplinary order against the respondent,

or to postpone judgement or to make a disciplinary order against the respondent.

10 If the committee decide upon a postponement, they then specify either a period for which judgement is postponed or a further committee meeting at which judgement will again be considered.

Procedure upon postponement

1 The solicitor to the GOC sends to the respondent not less than 6 weeks before the day fixed for the resumption of proceedings a notice containing:

   (a) the day, time and place set for the resumption of the proceedings

   (b) unless otherwise directed by the chairman of the committee, a letter inviting the respondent to furnish the names of character witnesses

   (c) an invitation to send any evidence relating to his conduct or any material facts which might have arisen since the original hearing. Any such information should reach the solicitor to the GOC no less than 3 weeks before the resumption of proceedings.

2 Any notice sent by the respondent after receipt of the above is passed on to the complainant for comment, and any such comment received by the solicitor to the GOC is supplied to the respondent.

3 At the resumed meeting, the solicitor to the GOC is invited to recall, for the information of the committee, the position at which the case stands.

4 The committee may now receive further oral or documentary evidence concerning the conduct of the respondent or any material facts that may have arisen since the original hearing.

5 The committee then considers their decision as before. Relating to resumed proceedings, any new charge which may be alleged against the respondent may be heard provided that the correct procedure has been followed and a decision made concerning all the charges. There is no question of the validity of the committee hearing even if the membership of the original enquiry and of the resumed proceedings differ. The chairman may postpone the resumed proceedings, either upon application of involved parties or at his own discretion, in which case the procedure for resumption is repeated.

It is the function of the Disciplinary Committee to decide whether the provision of the Opticians Act 1989 or the rules of the council have been contravened and to pass judgement accordingly. Any decisions made by the Disciplinary Committee are final, subject only to the right of appeal to the Judicial Committee of the Privy Council.

Jurisdiction

Under the terms of Section 17 of the Opticians Act 1989 the GOC has the power to erase from the register or list the name of any optician or corporate body following a disciplinary hearing if:

1 a registered optician is convicted by any court in the UK of any criminal offence which renders him or her unfit to have his/her name in the register
2 a registered optician is judged by the Disciplinary Committee to have been guilty of infamous conduct in any professional respect
3 a body corporate is convicted of an offence under the Opticians Act 1989 or is found guilty of aiding, abetting, counselling or procuring the commission of or inciting another person to commit such an offence
4 a body corporate no longer satisfies the criteria for enrolment as laid down in Section 9(2) of the Opticians Act 1989
5 a registered optician or body corporate contravenes or fails to comply with rules made by the GOC under Section 31 of the Opticians Act 1989 so as to render him/her or it unsuitable for continued registration
6 a registered optician or body corporate fails to ensure that optical appliances are fitted and supplied by or under the supervision of an appropriately qualified registered optician
7 the original entry for enrolment of the register or list was fraudulently or incorrectly made.

The changes in the legislation for registered opticians brought about by the Health and Social Security Act 1984 modified the jurisdiction of the GOC and the new General Optical Council Disciplinary Committee (Procedure) Rules 1985 contain the following as alternatives to an erasure order:

1 *A supervision order.* Under this new section the committee specify the period, not exceeding 12 months, during which the respondent's registration or enrolment shall be suspended.
2 *A penalty order.* As laid down in SI 1994/3327, and reviewed from time to time, any such order made under the regulations will specify the sum (currently not exceeding £1600 payable to the GOC) and the period within which the sum specified is to be paid.
3 *An erasure order or a suspension order* together with a penalty order.

The GOC has reviewed its disciplinary process and has issued for discussion a 'draft brief for legislative change' which it hopes will be adopted in the future. It has also introduced a fitness to practice code (see Chapter 13).

Disciplinary History of the GOC

Between the establishment of the Disciplinary Committee in 1960 and September 1982, there were 47 cases involving 101 charges against registered opticians or bodies corporate. On the basis of the hearings, 16 names were erased from the register or lists, and these may be broken down into:

- nine cases of conviction by UK courts of a serious offence
- four cases of infamous conduct in a professional respect, and

- three cases of contravention of the GOC regulations made under Section 25 of the Opticians Act 1958, relating to publicity.

The GOC has, in addition, made successful prosecutions against persons selling or supplying optical appliances contrary to the regulations under Section 21 of the Opticians Act 1958, limiting such acts to those qualified to be entered on the register or list.

More recently the GOC has seen an increase in activity and of 796 complaints made during the period 1994–1997, 26 cases were considered serious enough for referral to the Disciplinary Committee. In the year to 31 December 1999 a total of 195 complaints were received, 50 of which were referred to the full Investigating Committee for consideration. In the same period the Disciplinary Committee heard 10 cases (GOC annual report).

The types of cases brought before the GOC Disciplinary Committee are varied but examples from the three main areas are provided below.

1. Failure to detect and/or refer

There have been a number of cases in which it has been suggested that the individual failed to carry out a full investigation in view of the signs and symptoms of the individual patient presenting. The outcome of these varies and is dependent on the evidence presented at the time.

A number of factors will influence the decision. In one recent case a patient attended for a copy prescription and mentioned that a 'black arc' had appeared recently in 'the corner of the eye'. The practitioner failed to examine the eye simply checking vision through lenses on a test chart before issuing a copy prescription and therefore did not detect the detachment present. The committee felt that the actions constituted testing of sight as defined by the Opticians Act and accordingly the charge of serious professional misconduct was proved. The implications of this decision are wide reaching and could affect the sale of ready readers within a practice. If an optometrist assists a patient in the selection of the most appropriate ready reader and during the course of selection the patient mentions a symptom which may be considered as indicative of a more serious problem but the practitioner does not act the same conclusion as above could be reached.

In another case where the patient attended with symptoms of detachment and only a change of prescription was advised the practitioner concerned claimed that a referral letter was given to the patient and had a copy on file. As the referral letter, however, did not agree with the case records it was considered that it had been constructed at a later date when the details of the case were known. The practitioner was found guilty on counts of failure to carry out appropriate examination and failure to fulfil the requirements of referral.

At another hearing relating to failure to perform an adequate examination and failure to refer a different scenario developed. The patient was asked to return for a visual field examination a few days later but had a retinal detachment diagnosed by the general practitioner (GP) in the intervening period. The Disciplinary Committee found that the actions had fallen short of those required from a competent professional. It was felt that even without the additional information that would have been provided by a visual fields examination it was apparent that the patient was suffering from an injury, disease or abnormality and therefore should have been referred. It also felt, however, that although there was unacceptable professional conduct the circumstances were such that this fell short of serious professional misconduct. The lesson to be learned from this is that good records of patient examinations should be kept including symptoms and signs and that all tests that would be appropriate to the circumstances must be conducted.

In many of the cases the use of fields, tonometry and/or dilation are cited as being the accepted course of action following the signs or symptoms determined. Failure to carry out these tests may be considered as a lacking of professional competence. It is essential that this be borne in mind when assessing a patient with specific problems.

2. Publicity

As mentioned in the text this has become an area of considerable concern and one in which practitioners forget that the buck stops with them. A number of recent cases relate to situations in which advertisements have appeared suggesting one practitioner is better than others in a particular location. Terms such as 'premier optician' or 'leading optometrist' and descriptions such as 'finest range' or the 'best anywhere' should be avoided at all costs as these will undoubtedly be considered as unprofessional and lacking in substantiation.

3. Training and supervision

The role of the GOC in determining the suitability of training has been discussed earlier and there have been a number of occasions on which the approved institutions have had to revise aspects of their course to take on board GOC comments. The responsibility, however, also extends to the pre-registration year. Where it can be shown that a supervisor failed to adequately provide 'continuous personal supervision' then this would be considered as amounting to serious professional misconduct. A number of such cases have occurred recently.

Future Developments

The GOC has reviewed current statutory regulations and indicated a number of areas in which it would seek amendments. The suggested changes have been outlined in a document produced at the request of the council in 1999 (draft briefs for legislative change). The impetus for this revision came with the introduction of the Health Act 1999 that provided for regulatory bodies of professional groups to be granted greater freedom to introduce regulation. As yet these briefs have not been enacted although the GOC has submitted drafts for the introduction of compulsory CET and the direct supply of contact lenses.

Key points 1: Penalty orders which may be made by the GOC

1 Suspension of name from a register or list
2 Erasure of name from a register or list
3 A fine
4 A fine in combination with either of the other two orders

Key points 2: Complaints to the GOC about registered or enrolled opticians

Year	Complaints	Disciplinary hearings
1994	156	2
1995	198	8
1996	207	3
1997	235	13
1998	225	10
1999	195	10
2000	221	10

11

Referral and Case Records

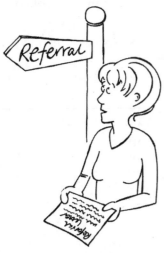

Patient referral is one of the most important functions of the optometrist in routine practice. Optometrists act as screeners to detect and send for further investigation those patients with ocular abnormalities and to monitor those patients identified with a condition that is not yet ready for treatment. That this screening and monitoring process is successful has been demonstrated by a number of articles in issues of the *British Journal of Ophthalmology* and other similar journals in which the referral service has been praised with special regard to glaucoma and diabetes. Further evidence for the success of the optometric profession in screening is provided by a diabetic study conducted by the Bristol Area Health Authority. Preliminary results suggest that the screening provided by optometrists in the area is so good that it is better than could normally be expected, and is better and more cost-effective than could be achieved by setting up specialized investigative services.

There are, therefore, very good reasons for the referral service within the general ophthalmic services, and, to aid in the smooth running of the service, there are certain legal requirements placed on the optometrist. Within the general ophthalmic services, under the terms of service as set out in SI 1986/975 and amended by SI 1989/1175, a patient should be referred to his or her general practitioner for the following specified conditions:

1 If there appears to be signs of injury, disease or abnormality in the eye or elsewhere which may require medical treatment.
2 If a satisfactory standard of vision is unlikely to be achieved even with corrective lenses.

In addition, a patient's general practitioner (GP) should be informed of the test results if the patient examined under the NHS has been diagnosed as:

1 diabetic
2 a glaucoma sufferer.

These regulations relate to the optometrist under contract to the National Health Service (NHS) and providing general ophthalmic services (GOS). Failure to comply with these rules could lead to disciplinary action by the Health Authority (HA) and, ultimately, withdrawal of the practitioner's name from the GOS lists.

In addition to the above regulations, the GOC have, in fulfillment of the duty laid on them under Section 31(5) of the Opticians Act 1989, published Rules Relating to Injury or Disease of the Eye, embodied in SI 1999/3267 (see Chapter 7). Under the terms of this instrument, where it appears to an optometrist that a patient is suffering from an injury or disease of the eye of which the patient's general medical practitioner may not be aware, the optometrist has two options:

1 refer the patient to the GP
2 monitor the patient and notify the GP if the condition is considered unlikely to deteriorate or to require treatment.

Failure to comply with this regulation could lead to a case being brought before the Disciplinary Committee of the GOC, and if negligence were proved, lead to erasure of the optometrist's name from the optician's register.

Guidance on the process of referral at one time was outlined in the GOCs now withdrawn N22. Since the withdrawal of this document no equivalent information has been produced although the College of Optometrist's guidelines do cover this area. The original GOC advice is still relevant in today's practice environment and it suggests the following steps should be taken when referring a patient to a registered medical practitioner:

1 The optometrist should advise the patient to consult his or her GP.
2 Wherever possible, a written report of the findings should be supplied, with an indication of the reasons for suspecting injury or disease. If a report is supplied, it should be on either headed notepaper or a standard acceptable form.
3 Should it appear that urgent action is required, every effort should be made to contact the GP immediately (e.g. by telephone). If it is not possible to contact the patient's GP then the patient should be sent, in the case of an emergency, to the nearest hospital accident and emergency unit with a letter on headed notepaper indicating the reason for referral. A copy of the letter with any further relevant information should be sent to the patient's GP.
4 If a patient is unwilling or refuses to consult the GP then the optometrist should record the grounds for the patient's refusal on the record card. The need for the patient to visit the GP should be stressed and if the patient still refuses they should be asked to sign the note on the record card as a disclaimer should the possibility of legal action arise at a future date.
5 The rules do not prohibit a registered optometrist from administering whatever services he/she may consider in the best interests of the patient in an emergency situation.

The GOC has defined the terms, 'injury or disease', as used initially in the Opticians Act 1958 and repeated in the Opticians Act 1989, to cover conditions which cause or are likely to cause detriment to health or sight, but excluding variations of refraction or normal changes due to age.

It is considered that, under SI 1999/3267, the optometrist transfers the authority for dealing with the patient to the GP upon referral. This has been interpreted as meaning that the GP should decide whether or not spectacles should be prescribed and be able to intercept if required.

In modern practice this is an unrealistic situation as patients may wait for up to 1 week for a non-urgent GP appointment and longer for a hospital consultant but can be supplied with spectacles within 1 h. As yet it appears that no case has been considered where an optometrist supplies spectacles and the GP then indicates that no spectacles should have been supplied.

In an emergency, for example, where a patient is unable to follow his occupation or is gravely inconvenienced without spectacles the optometrist has always been in a position to make the decision to supply spectacles provided that this is unlikely to prevent the patient from seeking further advice. It has been considered the responsibility of the GP to notify the optometrist if in his opinion the supply of spectacles would be inappropriate. If spectacles are supplied when a patient is referred then it should be made clear to the patient that the spectacles are supplied on a provisional basis and may need to be cancelled or returned if the GP feels that they should not be supplied.

General Referral Procedure

It is generally considered acceptable for the patient to take a letter by hand to the GP. This has certain advantages in that it is not dependent upon the postal services, and the problem of making appointments to coincide with the arrival of the letter is averted. Also the optometrist does not forget to send the letter and the GP does not forget receiving it! The disadvantages are that the patient may not actually visit the GP and also may be tempted to read the letter.

There is no legal or professional obligation to inform the patient of the contents of a referral letter unless it is requested under the terms of the Access to Health Records Act 1990 as updated by the Data Protection Act 1998. As a matter of courtesy, however, and to allay fears, it is normally better to inform the patient in general terms of the reasons for referral. This does not mean that the patient is given a diagnosis; under the terms of the NHS an optometrist is a detector of abnormality and not a diagnostician. There is obviously overlap between the two functions as recognized by the GOC referral rules of SI 1999/3267. It is better to indicate to the patient that a particular aspect is not normal rather than to give a definite named condition that may be incorrect or that may be subsequently refuted for reasons not apparent at the original examination.

Information-only referrals

Since the abolition of Form GOS 1 (used many years ago by GPs to refer patients to an optometrist), the optometrist has been expected, out of courtesy, to write to the GP in certain situations which would not constitute a referral. The situations are:

1 If a patient under the age of 16 years reports for an initial examination and, following the examination, no correction is given.
2 Where a patient reports for an eye examination and a further examination within 6 months is recommended.

There is no statutory duty to follow this and many GPs currently are overwhelmed with paperwork and therefore grateful not to receive such information.

There is however a statutory duty to notify the GP when a patient who has been diagnosed as suffering from either glaucoma or diabetes attends for a routine assessment. It has been suggested, following the new GOC rules on referral, the need to notify is present only when change occurs – this is not strictly correct and if this procedure is to be adopted it should be only after consultation with the local GPs and with their agreement.

Layout of referral letters

Referral to the patient's GP should be either by submission of an appropriate form, or on headed notepaper showing the practice address and the principal partners. Return letters from ophthalmologists to the referring optometrists vary from HA to HA. It was considered that if the appropriate form were used then a reply would be sent from the local ophthalmologist to the optometrist who referred. Recent work in Southampton has suggested that this is not always the case and that referral paperwork does not necessarily influence the frequency of response.

When using headed notepaper the letter should be dated and should begin with the patient's full name and address. It should contain details of history and symptoms, vision and visual correction with best acuities for distance and near, together with any previous acuities and the date recorded. The reasons for referral (e.g. motility problems, poor acuity, fundus abnormality) should be clearly stated. Finally the letter must be signed by the referring optometrist and a duplicate retained with the patient's record. A further copy of the letter should be sent to the GP for the patient's file. This last step is of great importance as a form of protection should there ever be the suggestion that no action was taken.

Case Records

This is an area of practice that receives far less attention than it deserves. It is the case record that can make or break a case of negligence. A sad finding from visiting different practices is the total inadequacy of many records. It is likely that most practitioners would not consider that they themselves are inadequate record keepers but this section, by outlining the bare minimum contents and demonstrating the essential elements of a record, may make them think again. The GOC have indicated that failure to keep acceptable and adequate records may be considered to constitute serious professional misconduct. Indeed there have been cases in which the GOC have made an erasure order on the basis of poor record keeping.

Record cards are intended to carry information pertinent to the patient's problems. They also act as a reminder to the practitioner of findings of an earlier examination and provide a means of evaluating change in basic measurements. The exact style of the record card is left to the individual practitioner. Records vary from simply blank cards to those providing enough space to include more detailed personal information such as the number of children the patient has, whether any children are going to university or taking up new jobs, particular hobbies and what the patient is hoping to do for a holiday.

Whatever the style of the record to be used, there are some basic points which should always be included.

Personal details

Name: There are few records that do not carry the patient's name. It is import-ant, however, that the full name is recorded and not just initials. From a filing point of view it can be an absolute nightmare trying to locate a Mr Jones in South Wales without the full name.

Address: This is also absolutely essential and should be updated whenever the patient points out a change.

Telephone number: It helps immensely if a patient can be reached by telephone during the day. For example, if something goes wrong with the promised job, you can advise the patient before he has to chase you.

Date of birth: The full date of birth is particularly necessary where, for example, father and son have the same names and live at the same address.

Date of examination: There is nothing more irritating for a patient who asks for the date of the last examination than to be told 'Oh, it was about 1983'. From a legal standpoint, the date of examination could be an import-ant factor in deciding whether or not a condition should have been noted at that time.

Occupation: It is usually necessary to know the patient's occupation. If glasses are prescribed for a specific occupation, they may prove totally unsuitable if the patient decides to change jobs.

GP's name and address: This information should be recorded for two reasons. First, it is needed for referral letters; secondly, if, as sometimes happens, a health clinic contacts the practice to ask for information about a patient, you can find out with whom you are dealing.

Hobbies: This information is necessary to help with the best choice of correction.

Clinical details from patient

Case history: Has the patient had an eye examination previously? If so, were spectacles prescribed and, if so, for what were they to be used? Has the patient ever had any eye injury or operation and, if so, what was its nature?

Symptoms: Why has the patient decided to visit an optometrist? Does he suffer from eye ache or headaches? When do the symptoms occur?

General health: Is the patient suffering from any general disorder or taking tablets, pills or other medication?

Family history: Is there any history of eye problems or of general health problems in the family?

Examination details

- Unaided vision
- retinoscopy

- subjective
- best corrected distance acuity
- distance muscle balance, etc.
- amplitude of accommodation
- near acuity
- near reading correction, if necessary
- near muscle balance
- external examination of the eyes.
- ophthalmoscopy: it is important that the case record shows that a full examination has been carried out. It may appear adequate to write 'NAD' in this section but this does not show that you actually examined any particular structure. A complete record should carry information such as: 'media clear, discs flat, cup/disc 0.2, fundus clear'; this at least shows that structures were examined
- supplementary tests carried out
- decision on patient disposal: this should include a copy of the referral note, if the patient is advised to visit his GP, or the patient's signature if such advice is rejected
- examiner's name
- dispensing details
  distance: Frame details, facial measurements and centration distance
  near: Frame details and centration distance
- costing: this comprises the charges and fees, and details of any deposit.

The above outline simply presents the basic information required; it does not offer a layout and it does not offer any advice on the relative importance of each category. Many optometrists will already use a case record that carries more information. In the present circumstances where the professional activity of optometrists is under scrutiny it is essential that every effort be made to protect one's clinical reputation. Complete and accurate case records are a simple and effective way of achieving this. A further reason for maintaining good records is the enactment of the Access to Health Records Act 1990 and the Data Protection Act 1998.

The Access to Health Records Act 1990

The Access to Health Records Act 1990 was laid before Parliament in July 1990 and came into force on 1 November 1991. It was drafted to establish a right of access to health records by the individuals to whom the records relate and to certain others and to provide for the correction of inaccurate health records. There have been some modifications introduced by the Data Protection Act 1998 that are included in the text.

Under the terms of the 1990 Act, a health record is defined as a record that:

1 consists of information relating to the physical or mental health of an individual who can be identified from that information or from that and other information in the possession of the holder of the record, and
2 have been made by or on behalf of a health professional in connection with the care of the individual.

The holder of the record is defined as any 'health professional' that is included in this meaning within the Data Protection Act 1998.

Right of access

Under Section 3 of the 1990 Act application for access to the record or to any part of the record may be made to the record holder by:

1 the patient
2 a person authorized in writing to make the application on the patient's behalf, for example, solicitor
3 where the record is held in England and Wales and the patient is a child, a person having parental responsibility for the patient
4 where the record is held in Scotland and the patient is a pupil, a parent or guardian of the patient
5 where the patient is incapable of managing his own affairs, any person appointed by a court to manage those affairs
6 where the patient has died, the patient's personal representative and any person who may have a claim arising out of the patient's death.

If an application is made to inspect the records, then providing the record was made more than 40 days before the application to view, the holder must allow inspection within 40 days of the date of the application.

In the case where details were entered on to the record within the 40 days preceding the application, inspection is required within 21 days of receipt of application. If requested the holder must supply a copy of the record or extract.

A fee cannot normally be made for access but the cost of copying and postage is recoverable. It is also a requirement that where information is expressed in terms that are not intelligible without explanation, a full explanation of the terms must accompany the copy or be furnished to the individual at inspection.

Section 3(6) allows for the situation in which:

1 the holder of the record is unable to identify the patient from the information included in the request for access, or
2 where the application is by an individual other than the patient the holder is unsure of the applicant's entitlement to make an application.

The holder is given 14 days from the date of the application to request the applicant to provide such further information as may be reasonably required. The time-scales are affected by this procedure such that the 40-day period discussed above relates to the new date when further information is supplied.

In an effort to protect further the interests of the patient and the practitioner, certain exclusions of access or partial exclusions of access are allowed for. These relate in the case of total exclusion to:

1 A child patient where the holder is not satisfied that the patient is capable of understanding the nature of the application.

2 A child patient where another individual has applied for access. The holder must be satisfied that the patient has consented to the making of the application, or that the patient is incapable of understanding the nature of the application but that granting of access would be in the patient's best interests.
3 In the case of a patient who has died, access to details will not be allowed where the record includes a note, made at the patient's request, that access should not be given if application were made.

In the case of partial exclusion these refer to:

1 Information likely to cause serious harm to the physical or mental health of the patient or any other individual.
2 Information relating to, or provided by, an individual other than the patient who could be identified from that information without prior consent of the individual.
3 Details entered on to a health record prior to commencement of the Access the Health Records Act (1 November 1991).
4 Information provided by the patient in the expectation that it would not be disclosed to any other individual without their authority.
5 Information obtained as a result of an examination that the patient consented to in the expectation that the information would not be disclosed to any other party.
6 Information that in the case of a deceased patient was not relevant to any claim which may arise out of the patient's death.

Correction of records

Section 6 of the Act allows for correction or amendment of health records. Where a person considers that any information contained in a health record to which they have access is incorrect, misleading or incomplete they may apply to the holder of the record for correction to be made. On such an application the holder shall:

1 if satisfied that the information is not correct, make the necessary correction
2 where not satisfied that the information is incorrect, make notes on the record of the applicant's comments regarding accuracy
3 in either case, without requiring a fee, supply the applicant with a copy of the correction or note.

It is important to note that the term 'information' when relating to a health record includes any expression of opinion about the patient.

The Data Protection Act 1998 has had only a minor effect on the conditions introduced by the Access to Health Records Act 1990 and is discussed in more detail in Chapter 19.

Key points 1: Referral/notification under NHS terms of service

1 Where there appears to be signs of injury disease or abnormality in the eye or elsewhere
2 If a satisfactory standard of vision is unlikely to be achieved even with corrective lenses
3 Where a patient has been diagnosed as diabetic
4 Where a patient has been diagnosed as a glaucoma sufferer

Key points 2: Legislation relating to case records

1 The Data Protection Act 1984
2 The Access to Health Records Act 1990
3 The Data Protection Act 1998

12

The Law Relating to the Use of Drugs

Medicines Act 1968

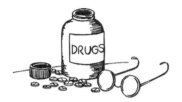

In January 1978, the government published the long-awaited statutory instruments bringing into force Part III of the Medicines Act 1968, and announced that the 'appointed day' would be 1 February 1978. Such was the extent of the change made in these orders that a supplementary order had to be made later, postponing certain of the provisions for 6 months. This delay was to give the pharmaceutical industry and the profession of pharmacy sufficient time to come to terms with the new regulations concerning the sale and supply of some drugs.

Not least to be affected by the new regulations was the optometrist, who gained the right to supply, as well as use, an even greater range of drugs than before. In order fully to understand the provisions relating to the use of drugs by optometrists, it is necessary first to summarize briefly the various parts of the Medicines Act 1968 and then look at the various subsequent orders made.

The Medicines Act 1968, covering as it does such a wide range of activities concerned with the production and supply of medicines, is no mean document and is divided into eight parts, containing in all 136 sections and eight schedules. Schedules 5–8 list all the previous enactments to be repealed or amended with the coming into force of the main Act.

Part I of the Medicines Act 1968 deals with administration; Section 2 sets up the Medicines Commission and Committees under it. The Medicines Commission consists of not fewer than eight members, representing the following 'activities' – medicine, veterinary medicine, pharmacy, pharmaceutical industry and chemistry.

The 45 sections of Part II deal with the licensing of the manufacture, import, export and wholesale of medicinal products. No person may manufacture or assemble or wholesale any product unless he has a licence to do so. Such a 'blanket' law is, of course, subject to many exemptions. For example, it would be time consuming for a pharmacist to obtain a licence every time he wished to make a particular prescription for a particular patient and he is thus exempted from the necessity of obtaining a licence for manufacture under these conditions. There are further exemptions for doctors, dentists, veterinary practitioners, nurses and midwives. There are also exemptions for herbal remedies and there were transitional exemptions for products which were on the market on the appointed day.

The most important sections as far as the optometrist is concerned are included in Part III, which deals with the sale or supply of medicinal products. In order to understand the various orders introduced in February 1978, it is necessary to look at certain sections of this part in detail.

Section 51 allowed the minister to set up a 'General Sale List' (GSL) of drugs which can be reasonably sold without the supervision of a pharmacist. Section 53 allows for certain drugs to be sold by automatic machine (i.e. an automatic machine section to the GSL).

All drugs not on this list may be sold only by 'a person lawfully conducting a retail pharmacy business' or on premises registered as a pharmacy and under the supervision of a pharmacist (Section 52). This restriction previously was applied by including a substance in Part I of the Poisons List, when sale could be made only by an 'authorized seller of poisons' (note the change in title). Now, paradoxically, it is the non-inclusion of a substance in a list that brings this restriction into force. Since it allows certain substances to be sold other than at a pharmacy even if they are not included on a GSL, a very important rider to the regulation states 'subject to any exemption conferred by or under this part of the Act'. This rider is included in Section 52 and several other sections of the Act.

Sections 53 and 54 lay down the conditions under which GSL substances may be sold, and Sections 55–57 lay down broad exemptions from Section 52.

Further restrictions are imposed under Section 58 that allows for another list of medicinal substances called the 'Prescription Only List' to be set up. Under Subsection (2), medicines on the Prescription Only List can be supplied only in accordance with a prescription issued by an 'appropriate practitioner' (a term defined in subsection (1) as being doctors, dentists or veterinarians). The remainder of Section 58 deals with exemptions from this restriction, subject to conditions that may be defined in the relevant orders.

The rest of Part III deals with other conditions concerning the sale or supply of medicinal substances and need not concern us here (especially Section 67, which deals with fines and imprisonment for contravening Sections 52 and 58).

Parts IV, V, VI, VII and VIII deal with pharmacies, containers, promotion of sales, official publications and miscellaneous provisions, respectively.

Nowhere in the Act are specific medicinal substances listed. The inclusion of substances in the GSL or in the Prescription Only List is the subject of the various orders brought into effect on 1 February 1978 and subsequently revised. Principal among these are the GSL and the Prescription Only List.

General Sale List

The GSL is a list of human and veterinary drugs defined by Section 51 of the Medicines Act and contains the common (and some not so common) medicinal substances which can be sold other than at a pharmacy. Provided that Section 53 is complied with, an ophthalmic optician may sell any substance on the GSL.

Schedule 6 of the order (SI 1977/2129) however, lists medicinal products that are not on the GSL and includes products marketed as medicinal eye drops or eye ointments. Thus all medicinal eye drops, whether for human or for animal use, are not on general sale even though the active principle may be included in the list.

Prescription Only Medicines List

It will surprise optometrists to find that many of the drugs commonly in use by them are included in Schedule 1 of the prescription only medicines (POM) List. Even though the schedule exempts many of these drugs from the class of prescription only when they are applied externally, local ophthalmic use is often excluded from the exemption. For example, atropine is prescription only unless applied externally by a route other than to the eye.

It can be seen that eye drops and eye ointment have been singled out for special attention both in their exclusion from the GSL and in the external application exemption from the POM list.

Pharmacy List

This is a catch all list and any preparation that does not appear on the GSL or the POM lists is automatically covered by the Pharmacy List as defined by Section 52 of the Medicines Act. All drugs included on this list would normally be sold or supplied from a registered pharmacy under the supervision of a registered pharmacist. In the case of a pharmacy medicine that is an eye drop or ointment it can be used and supplied by an optometrist – supply being by way of a signed order for presentation to a pharmacist.

Initially published under the terms of the Medicines (Prescription only) Order 1977/No. 2127, as amended by The Medicines (Prescription only) Order Amendment No. 2 1978/No. 287, Schedule 4 Part I 5(2), subsequently revised by SI 1983/1212 and again by SI 1989/1852, as Schedule 3(l) 5 and 6 and by SI 1997/1830 schedule 5 part 1, is a list of exemptions from Section 58(2) – (the section by which a prescription is required before drugs on the list can be supplied). Paragraph 5 allows pharmacists to supply certain specified eye drops or ointments subject to the presentation of an order signed by a registered optometrist. Paragraph 6 allows optometrists to supply the same drugs in the course of their professional practice or in an emergency. The drugs, if supply is covered by this exemption, will be found in Table 12.1. Interestingly enough this schedule only gives exemption from Section 58, it does not give exemption from Section 52 (supply only by a pharmacist). The exemption from this latter section is given in another completely separate order – the Medicines (Pharmacy and General Sale – Exemption) Order 1977 as amended by SI 1978/No. 988, and SI 1980/1924 – which exempts optometrists from the requirements of Section 52 for the same drugs in the schedule. This order also provides a general, transitional exemption from Section 52 for products that could have been supplied lawfully before the appointed day. This exemption lasted for 2 years.

One further order, the Medicines (Sale or Supply) (Miscellaneous Provisions) Regulations 1977, SI 1977/2132, as amended by SI 1978/989 and subsequently included in SI 1980/1923, allows the optometrist to obtain and use a further range of drugs. The particular regulation relates to wholesale dealing, which is defined in the Medicines Act 1968 as being 'supply to a person for retail sale, or for administering to a human being in the course of a business carried on by him'. Since this order does not give exemption from Section 52, only the latter purpose is catered for; i.e. optometrists may use these drugs in their practice but must not supply them to their

Table 12.1 Commonly used ophthalmic drugs and their legal classification

Drug	Legal class	Optometrist Uses	Supplies
Adrenaline (in eye drop form)	P	y	n
Adrenaline acid tartrate (in eye drop form)	P	y	n
Adrenaline hydrochloride (in eye drop form)	P	y	n
Amethocaine hydrochloride	POM	y	n
Antazoline (upto 1%)	P	y	y
Artificial tears	P	y	y
Atropine sulphate	POM	y	y
Bethanechol chloride (n/a)	POM	y	y
Carbachol	POM	y	y
Chloramphenicol drops (<0.5%)	POM	y	y
Chloramphenicol ointment (<1%)	POM	y	y
Cyclopentolate hydrochloride	POM	y	y
Dibromopropamidine isethionate (Brolene ointment)	P	y	y
Ephedrine (in eye drop form)	P	y	n
Ephedrine hydrochloride (eye drop form)(n/a)	P	y	n
Ephedrine sulphate (eye drop form) (n/a)	P	y	n
Fluorescein sodium	P	y	y
Framycetin sulphate	POM	y	n
Homatropine hydrobromide	POM	y	y
Hyoscine hydrobromide (n/a)	POM		y
Hypromellose	P	y	y
Lignocaine hydrochloride	POM	y	n
Mafenide propionate (<5%)	P	y	y
Naphazoline hydrochloride (<0.015%)	P	y	y
Naphazoline hydrochloride (>0.015%)	POM	y	n
Oxybuprocaine hydrochloride (Benoxinate)	POM	y	n
Oxyphenbutazone ointment (n/a)	POM	y	n
Phenylephrine hydrochloride	P	y	y
Physostigmine sulphate (n/a)	POM	y	y
Pilocarpine hydrochloride	POM	y	y
Pilocarpine nitrate	POM	y	y
Propamidine isethionate (Brolene eye drops)	P	y	y
Proxymetacaine hydrochloride	POM	y	n
Sodium chromoglycate	P	y	y
Sodium chromoglycate	POM	n	n
Sulphacetamide sodium (up to 30%)(n/a)	POM	y	y
Thymoxamine hydrochloride (n/a)	POM	y	n
Tropicamide	POM	y	y
Xylometazoline (Otrivine)	P	y	y
Zinc sulphate			

P: pharmacy medicines; y: yes; n: no.

patients. Most of the drugs in this order are the local anaesthetics that should never be given to patients for their own use in any situation. The commonly used ophthalmic preparations and their legal classification are shown in Table 12.1. Further details of individual drugs listed can be found in 'The Optometrists Formulary' published by the College of Optometrists (1998).

In specific emergency circumstances, optometrists may decide that the best course of action for the patient is to supply them directly with exempted POM or ophthalmic pharmacy only medicinal products. In such a case, the optometrist may re-label pre-packed preparations without holding a licence for assembly. This position has been achieved through the GOC's application for a general exemption for registered opticians under the requirements of Article 2 of the Medicines (Exemptions from Licences) (Assembly) Order 1979 No. 114. The exemption does not apply to contact lens fluids and a separate individual exemption would be needed for this situation under the requirements of Medicines (Contact Lens Fluids and Other Substances) (Exemption from Licences) Order 1979 No. 1585.

If re-labelling is undertaken by the optometrist, then to meet the labelling regulations for a dispensed medicinal product, the following information, written in indelible ink, is required on the product:

1 the name of the patient
2 the directions for use
3 the words 'Keep out of reach of children'
4 the phrase 'For external use only'
5 the date of supply
6 the name and address of the supplying optometrist.

Although the Medicines Act 1968 is wide ranging in its effects, it is not the only Act that affects the sale and supply of drugs. So-called 'controlled drugs' are covered by the Misuse of Drugs Act 1971. All standard eye preparations of cocaine come under this Act and hence cannot be used by an optometrist.

Contact lens care products underwent a change in 1995 and prior to this date they were required to have a product licence from the Medicines Control Agency. Subsequent to this date all contact lens care products are now required to have a CE marking and number. Should an optometrist wish to re-label a contact lens care product the Medical Devices Agency would be able to provide the appropriate information.

It can be seen that the effect of the legislation was to increase the range of drugs that the optometrist may use and supply. Apart from in an emergency, the use or supply of drugs must be in line with the practice of the profession of optometry as defined in the Opticians Act 1989 or laid down by the GOC. Nothing in the 1968 Act has changed the restrictions concerning treatment of adverse ocular conditions.

Prescription Writing

In the normal course of practice, two situations may arise concerning the supply of drugs for use in the practice, in which case two courses are open.

In the first situation, either the practitioner may write out a signed order or, in the case of a 'poison' (as defined in the Medicines Act) which is still available for use in the practice, he may sign the poisons register.

As an example the format for a signed order for physostigmine is

Name of practitioner, qualifications   Address of practitioner
Ophthalmic optician/optometrist   Date
Please supply, for use in my practice,
X single units (minims) physostigmine salicylate BP 0.25%
Signature of practitioner

The other situation that may arise concerns the use of a prescription to supply a substance such as atropine for instillation by the patient at home prior to an appointment for visual examination. In this second situation the format for the signed order for supply is

Name of practitioner, qualifications   Address of practitioner
Ophthalmic optician/optometrist
Name of patient (and age if under 14 years)
Address of patient
Name and formula of preparation and strength
Quantity to be supplied
Labelling instructions
Signature of practitioner   Date

Emergency Treatment and Supply

It is unlikely that an optometrist will be involved in the emergency treatment of a patient. However, it is well known that patients do not confine themselves to requiring assistance at convenient times. If a patient requires assistance and no medical practitioner is readily available, no hospital casualty department is accessible, and no pharmacy open in the near vicinity, it may be that such a situation arises. In any case where such action is taken by a registered optometrist, the patient must be advised to contact their general practitioner at their earliest convenience and the optometrist must make every effort to supply the practitioner with the details of the background to the action and the action taken. As O'Connor Davies (1978) put it, 'It should be remembered that every emergency treatment or direct supply by the optometrist must be justified in the light of special and un-usual circumstances prevailing in that particular case. The patient's interests must be paramount and the optometrist must always conform to the relevant regulations as laid down by the Medicines Act and subsequent statutory instruments.'

The Crown Report

Following on from the publication of the Department of Health's white paper 'Primary Care: Delivering the Future' (1996) a Review of Prescribing, Supply and Administration of Medicines Team was established in 1997.

The aims of the review team were to:

1 develop a framework to determine in what circumstances health professionals could undertake new roles with regard to the prescribing, supply and administration of medicines
2 consider the implications for legislation and professional training.

The constraints for change were that:

1 any changes to existing roles must at the very least maintain, and preferably enhance, patient safety
2 changes need to be cost-effective
3 there should be demonstrable benefits to patient care.

An interim report from the team 'Review of Prescribing, supply and administration of medicines – a report on the supply and administration of medicines under Group Protocols' was published in 1998. The Final report in 1999.

The outcome of the report is a series of recommendations to take forward prescribing of medicines. Two new classes of prescriber are suggested:

1 Independent who would assess patients with undiagnosed conditions, make a diagnosis and be responsible for decisions about the clinical management required including prescribing.
2 Dependent who would be responsible for the continuing care of a patient who had been assessed by an independent prescriber.

Optometrists appear in the list of professions recommended for inclusion as independent prescribers. The report states 'Optometrists' expertise relating to the eye and visual system, coupled with the use of specialized diagnostic instruments, is the basis of the care they provide in the community, including domiciliary visits. Having established a diagnosis, prescribing would allow them to provide effective treatment for emergency eye conditions and non-sight threatening eye conditions.'

While there is no current legislation enabling optometrists to undertake independent prescribing the recognition provided by this report should lead to such developments in the foreseeable future.

Key points 1: Sale and supply of drugs are controlled by

1 GSL
2 POM List
3 Pharmacy List
4 Misuse of Drugs Act 1971

13

Professional Ethics and Disciplinary Measures within the Profession

General Ethics

Before 1988, there were two major sources of ethical and professional guidance; the one produced by the professional body the British College of Optometrists (BCO) and the other by the statutory body, the General Optical Council (GOC), in support of its regulations. Notice N22 however, published in March 1987 was the last guidance to be issued by the GOC, and after much discussion it was decided in 1988 to withdraw the Notice, and for future cases in which professional conduct was under review to use a 'peer group' view.

The effect of withdrawal of N22 was to place greater demands on the guidelines of The College of Optometrists and in order to meet the demands and fully to take the place of N22 a complete revision was undertaken resulting in the 1991 Publication of Guidance. These guidelines were reviewed by other optical organizations such as Federation of Ophthalmic and Dispensing Opticians (FODO), Federation of Independent British Optometrists and the Association of Optometrists before publication and amended to take account of points raised where this was a general opinion. The result of this activity was guidance that took account of the views of all major optometric organizations and represented a consensus of opinion.

Although the GOC has withdrawn guidance it remains the statutory body for optometric practice and therefore may take action against any registered optometrist where it feels that statutory requirements have not been met. The College of Optometrists, on the other hand, is a professional organization the aim of which is to maintain, for the public benefit, the highest possible standard of professional competence and conduct and as such it can only take action against its own members. Although the GOC will take note of the College of Optometrists guidance in any action taken against a practitioner both it and the Courts could override the college view if it were to be shown to differ from that of the reasonably competent 'average' practitioner under similar circumstances.

Due to legislative changes and consumer attitudes the 1991 Guidelines became out of date and in 1997 the College of Optometrists released details of updated guidance specifically on the routine eye examination. The update however was in a different format to previous guidance and provided advice on BEST practice. While this was very laudable and provided a target to which every practitioner could aspire and self-assess it was not a peer view of current practice. The result was to create friction within the profession and the college agreed to review the guidelines. The review is now completed and due for issue in 2001.

The 1991 code of ethics of the College of Optometrists still forms the basis for the professional conduct of optometrists and all fellows and members of the college are required to subscribe to it. The code states:

> An optometrist shall always place the welfare of the patient before all other considerations, and shall behave in a proper manner towards professional colleagues and shall not bring them or the profession into disrepute.

The guidance that the college issues represents its view of how the code of ethics should be interpreted by fellows and members in their professional lives and currently covers six main areas:

1 *Professional integrity:* It is the overriding and continuing responsibility of all practitioners to place the welfare of their patients before all other considerations, and to apply to each patient the full extent of their knowledge and skill and to maintain and develop professional competence throughout their professional life.
2 *Practitioner/patient relationship:* The relationship between practitioners and patients is an individual one and depends on mutual trust. Practitioners should do everything to promote their patients' confidence in them and in the profession as a whole and have a duty to ensure as far as possible that patients understand the actions and outcomes of their eye examination.
3 *Professional relationships:* It is contrary to the interests of patients that any ill feeling should be engendered, for whatever reason, between an optometrist and other members of the optometric or other health care professions. Scrupulous care should be taken to observe professional courtesies at all times, and to resolve, quickly and amicably, any difficulties, which arise. The optometrist has a duty to do everything possible to promote and preserve colleagues' and other health care professionals' confidence in himself and in the profession as a whole.
4 *Delegation:* The optometrist has a duty to ensure that the patient receives the same standard of clinical care whether or not he delegates any part of the eye examination, and to satisfy himself as to the competence and suitability of the person to perform the part being delegated.
5 *The routine eye examination:* The optometrist has a duty to carry out whatever tests are necessary to determine the patient's needs for vision care as to both the sight test and health. The exact format and content will be determined by the practitioner's professional judgement and the minimum legal requirements.
6 *Contact lens practice:* This covers the whole range of contact lens practice to which the fundamental principles of professional conduct apply in full. An optometrist has a duty to ensure that he always works within his limit of clinical competency when engaging in specialist areas of contact lens practice.

To support these six areas, the college has published an extensive set of guidelines that are issued to all fellows and members and that will from time to time be amended to take account of legislative and professional changes. All fellows and members agree to abide by these annually when they sign on renewal of their association with the college.

The following provides a brief outline of the areas covered within the guidelines but should not be considered as a comprehensive review. Anyone who would like a copy of the full guidelines should contact the College of Optometrists.

Outline of BCO Guidelines

The guidelines are in two parts the first covering ethics the second covering clinical practice.

Ethics

Professional integrity

The concept of professional integrity is the foundation of the whole code of ethics and guidelines and is concerned with the duty to put the interests of the patient first in all circumstances. The college has considered that to fulfil this the practitioner must:

1 maintain a high standard of competence and be aware of any limitations in their knowledge
2 maintain and expand their professional skills and knowledge by attending regular refresher courses
3 if intending to practise in specialist areas be sure that they have the necessary training and skills
4 ensure that they are adequately covered by indemnity insurance to protect the patient's interests.

The eye examination

The eye examination is considered to be the primary optometric function, the purpose of which is to determine the patient's needs in all aspects of vision care. Changes in the law brought about by the Sight Testing (Examination and Prescription) Regulations 1989 mean that a statutory duty of care is placed upon optometrists such that whenever a person's sight is tested within the meaning of Section 24 as defined by Section 36(2) of the Opticians Act 1989, a full eye examination must be carried out.

The content of an eye examination will vary depending upon the individual needs of the patient and the guidelines provide a basic outline of the tests that could be included. In the final analysis it is expected that the examination given must be such as to:

1 detect ocular abnormality
2 allow the prescribing of functional corrections for defects of sight
3 determine the need for remedial vision training where appropriate
4 provide advice to the patient on all aspects of visual efficiency.

Guidance issued in 2001 provides information on specialist forms of the examination and advice is therefore found in respect of examinations carried out on:

- patients with diabetes mellitus
- patients at risk from primary open angle glaucoma
- the younger child
- the older person
- domiciliary visits.

In all of the above cases the College recognizes that in co-management schemes the locally agreed protocols governing the scheme will take precedence over the guidance offered by the College.

Within the clinical practice section the College also offers guidance on:

- patient records
- referrals/notifications
- prescriptions
- sale and supply of optical appliances and standards
- the use of drugs in optometric practice.

Contact lens practice

This area of practice has seen rapid expansion and redevelopment and, therefore, requires a more dynamic guideline that can be rapidly amended to take account of new developments in product and technique. The guidelines outline equipment needs and clinical procedures including the need for effective after-care arrangements.

The GOC Rules on specifications for contact lenses are discussed and advice given to enable the practitioner to apply these rules to serve the best interests of their patients. The guidance covers both issue and receipt of specifications and cases of ongoing care.

Optometrists acting against the guidelines

This comprehensive set of guidelines is aimed at maintaining the high standard of patient care that is expected within the UK by all patients. The steps that may be taken by the GOC to investigate and discipline an optometrist for alleged offences have been outlined in Chapter 10. Ultimately, the GOC may erase a practitioner's name from the register and, therefore, prevent them from practising. The college has a more flexible approach to the problem, and although a formal investigation and disciplinary procedure can be undertaken, this is rarely required.

The initial step for the College of Optometrists following a complaint is for the College Professional Adviser to contact the individuals concerned, and wherever possible, to resolve the problem. If it is considered that the complaint is such that the GOC should investigate, then the college will formally pass the complaint over. If the complaint is such that it is not a GOC matter and also cannot be resolved by the Professional Adviser process the matter would be referred to the College Investigation Committee for formal consideration.

If after consideration the Investigating Committee feel that the matter is serious enough to warrant consideration of Serious Professional Misconduct it will be referred to the Disciplinary Committee. If such a case is proven the Disciplinary Committee may impose one of the following penalties on the respondent:

- expulsion from the college
- suspension from membership of the college for a fixed period or for a period expiring on a fixed date
- an undertaking that a specific action will be taken in a specified time
- a reprimand either orally or in writing

The College of Optometrists has attempted to interpret existing regulations and to provide guidance for optometric practice, but it is the GOC who have the more effective powers available. The college will take, and indeed in the past has taken steps to remove or suspend individuals from membership, but the GOC alone can prevent an optometrist from practising.

Fitness to practice procedures

The GOC decided in 1997 that there were cases in which the Investigating Committee did not wish to refer the practitioner to the Disciplinary Committee but that there was concern about specific aspects of the practitioner's professional practice. To overcome this an informal and voluntary procedure for dealing with fitness to practice was introduced in conjunction with the College of Optometrists. The role of the college is to provide support and advice for the practitioner to help to avoid similar problems in the future.

The college suggests the benefits of this fitness to practice procedure from the optometrist's perspective are:

1 The practitioner has the opportunity to review his or her actions in discussion with peers, with the sole objective of highlighting problem areas and avoiding future difficulties.
2 The practitioner is given positive and constructive help, in a non-confrontational setting.
3 Where appropriate, practical training is arranged or courses recommended, to help enhance skills for future practice.

It suggests from the GOCs perspective:

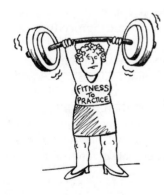

1 The GOC can tackle matters of concern that are not necessarily appropriate for the statutory disciplinary process.
2 Public protection is safeguarded, since perceived deficiencies in practice are addressed.

The process involved is simple and straightforward. After receiving details from the GOC the college invites the practitioner concerned to attend the college to discuss the professional and clinical aspects of the case with the Professional Adviser and the Secretary. The advice and any recommendations resulting from the interview are ratified by the College's Professional

Conduct Committee and confirmed in writing to the practitioner. The college monitors implementation of any recommended action and once a satisfactory outcome has been achieved a report is made to the GOC indicating a satisfactory conclusion.

The college website indicates that as of the 22/12/2000, 32 cases had been dealt with through this procedure. Some examples of the types of cases reviewed have appeared in the optical press (Taylor and Edwards, 1998).

AOP Advice on Content of the Eye Examination

More recently the issue of content of an eye examination has been raised with respect to the NHS sight test. The Association of Optometrists has issued a document 'The eye examination and related matters' (1999) as a guidance and consultation document. The main purpose of the document was an attempt to clarify the end point of an examination and to explain the circumstances under which a supplementary fee may be charged to the patient in the course of a sight test.

In an attempt to 'draw lines' the advice recommends that a sight test should be viewed as being of two main components the first containing all the tests needed to determine the need for referral, the second to refine the referral. It has been suggested that at the point at which an abnormality is noted the patient could be given the option of referral or the option of paying for additional tests which by refining the data could determine the nature of the abnormality. The benefits of supplementary testing are immediate confirmation of a problem should one exist and therefore reduction in the anxiety that may be induced through not knowing the outcome and waiting for a hospital consultation. This is obviously a very fine line and should a patient not be able to pay and therefore tests not be completed the service they would be getting would not be of the expected standard. Similarly if a practitioner stopped at a point which did not determine the urgency for referral and the patient suffered long-term problems as a result of a poor referral it may be that the patient could take action against the practitioner.

Key points 1: College of Optometry guidance covers

1 Professional integrity
2 Practitioner/patient relationship
3 Professional relationships
4 Delegation
5 The routine eye examination
6 Contact lens practice

Key points 2: Perceived benefits of the fitness to practice procedure

1 Helps practitioners to review their actions and highlight problem areas
2 Practitioners receive positive and constructive help
3 Training is arranged if appropriate/required
4 Perceived deficiencies are addressed safeguarding public protection
5 The GOC can deal with matters that would not fall within the statutory disciplinary process

---

It is often found that in practice patients ask the standards of vision required for various occupations. There is some difficulty in obtaining the information *en masse* and as a guide some of the more commonly requested requirements are therefore laid out below.

Motor Vehicle Driving Licence

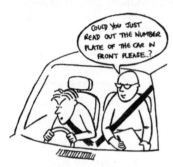

Applicants for a licence are required to meet the conditions laid down in the Motor Vehicles (Driving Licences) Regulations (SI 1981/952). They must be able to read, in good daylight (with the aid of glasses if worn), a registration mark fixed to a motor vehicle at a distance of 75 ft in the case of a registration mark containing letters and figures 3.5 in. high or at a distance of 67 ft (20.5 m) in the case of a registration mark containing letters and figures 3.125 in. high. An offence is committed by anyone who drives at any time with eyesight that does not meet this standard under Section 96 of the Road Traffic Act 1988. A further offence is now committed by a licence holder who fails to notify the Licensing Centre when eyesight falls below this standard or when specifically advised that it is likely to fall below that standard. The obligation to notify disabilities to the Licensing Centre extends in the case of eyesight, to any other defects of vision which affect, or may in time affect, a driver's ability to drive safely.

In practice there is no precise Snellen equivalent to the number plate standard. It has been suggested that the nearest equivalent on a standard test chart is between 6/9 and 6/12 (Drasdo and Haggerty, 1981) but this is not a statutory standard.

Large Goods Vehicles and Passenger-carrying Vehicles Driving Licences

Applicants are required to reach an uncorrected standard of visual acuity of 6/60 in each eye and have a corrected acuity of at least 6/9 in the better eye and 6/12 in the poorer eye. If their performance is below this standard then they should be referred to an ophthalmologist for advice as to whether they should be allowed to drive. Those drivers who can reach this standard only with spectacles should always carry a spare pair. (The previous recommendations for visual acuity did not mention any minimum standard without glasses.)

Vocational licences are still issued to contact lens wearers and to patients who have had a cataract extraction, and to pseudophakic patients provided that they can meet the uncorrected standard of static acuity of 6/60 in each eye and other requirements laid down above.

The regulations now prohibit uniocular drivers from being granted a license to drive passenger-carrying vehicles or large goods vehicles. There is however no examination requirement for anyone applying for a provisional license although all applicants are asked to indicate that they have no visual problems.

Student and Private Pilot's Licences

1 Full and normal field of vision.
2 A visual acuity of at least 6/12 (20/40; 0.5) in each eye separately with or without correcting glasses. In the case of a correction over ±5.00 D a specialist's opinion is required.
3 A record should be made of any degree of heterophoria present.
4 The candidate should be able to read Jaeger No. 3 at 30–50 cm or its equivalent at the same distance, with each eye separately, allowing correcting lenses to be worn if it is the usual habit of the candidate to wear such lenses.
5 Contact lenses may be used provided binocular vision is correctable to at least 6/12. Any person wishing to use contact lenses should have a wearing time of several hours a day and should have been wearing lenses for at least 6 months. A specialist's report should be submitted.
6 Monocular candidates should be referred to the Civil Aviation Authority, Medical Department, CAA House, Kingsway, London WC2B 6TE.
7 If the Ishihara test shows defective colour vision then the Giles/Archer or Holmes–Wright lantern test must be carried out.

Any problems encountered when confronted by a prospective candidate for a private pilot's licence should be directed to the Civil Aviation Authority (CAA).

Professional Pilots Licences

The requirements for professional pilot's licences (i.e. ALTP, SCPL and CPL) are:

1 There should be no acute or chronic disease in either eye or adnexae.
2 The fields of vision should be normal.
3 A visual acuity of at least 6/9 (20/30; 0.7) in each eye separately, with or without correcting glasses. If correcting glasses are required, the unaided vision must not be less than 6/60 (20/200; 0.1) and the refractive error must not exceed ±3.00 D (equivalent spherical error); in addition, a spare pair of suitable lenses should always be carried. In such cases the medical certificate will bear an endorsement noting the requirement to wear correcting glasses.
4 Any degree of heterophoria found in the test should be noted in the candidate's medical record (hyperphoria greater than 1.5 prism D or esophoria greater than 6 prism D is not normally accepted).
5 Candidates are required to have accommodation which permits them to read the Faculty of Ophthalmology reading chart N5 or its equivalent at a distance of 30–50 cm with each eye separately, with or without correcting glasses.

6 The wearing of contact lenses is not permitted in professional pilots.
7 The candidate is required to have normal colour vision perception as tested by Ishihara pseudo-isochromatic plates in good daylight; alternatively, he must be able to recognize the colours of signal red, signal green and white using the large and medium apertures of a Giles/Archer lantern at a distance of 20 ft in a darkened room after 10 mm of dark adaptation.
8 The prescription of corrections for both near and distance vision should be notified.

Merchant Shipping

Merchant shipping sight test standards are laid down in Notice M 1061. The regulation is in two sections.

Section 1 applies to young persons and new entrants about to embark on a career in the fishing industry or on merchant navy vessels:

1 Before embarking on a sea-going career in a desk capacity every young person should undergo a thorough examination in both form and colour vision by an ophthalmologist.
2 A letter test is carried out using Snellen charts, the subject being required to read correctly down to and including line 7 with the better eye and down to and including line 6 with the other eye. This should relate to acuities of 6/6 and 6/7.5.
3 A lantern test is carried out in a darkened room. A series of red, white or green lights are shown either singly through a large aperture or two at a time through small apertures side by side. The candidate is required to name the colours correctly as they appear.
4 During the examination candidates will not be allowed to wear spectacles, contact lenses or glasses of any kind or any other artificial aid to vision. Treatment designed to improve vision temporarily should not be undertaken shortly before the test.

Section 2 applies to candidates for Department of Trade sight tests for a first certificate of competency or higher certificate and voluntary applicants for the sight test other than new entrants to the merchant navy or fishing industry. The sight test may be taken with or without aids (conventional spectacles or contact lenses) at the candidate's option, but different requirements apply to each option.

1 If aids are used:
  (a) the letter test is first carried out without the aids, and the requirement is to read down to and including line 5 with the better eye and down to and including line 3 with the other eye
  (b) the test is repeated with the aids, the requirement being to read correctly down to and including line 7 with the better eye and down to and including line 6 with the other eye.
2 If the sight test is carried out without aids then the applicant will be required to read down to and including line 7 with the better eye and down to and including line 6 with the other eye.
3 Candidates who have failed a test without aids may apply to retake the test locally with aids after a period of not less than 1 month.

4 Candidates who have failed a test when not using aids may be re-examined locally without aids after a period of 1 month.

Metropolitan Police Force

The requirement for entry as a constable in the Metropolitan Police is that the acuity with or without spectacles is at least 6/6 in the good eye and 6/12 in the poorer eye, with a binocular acuity of 6/6 and a minimum unaided vision in each eye of 6/18. The applicant is also required to pass the fourteenth edition of the Ishihara test plates for colour vision or at least show the 'ability to distinguish the principal colours'. The regulations for other police forces across the UK do vary and it would be necessary to contact the local police information office to identify requirements in a particular area.

British Railways

This group may be divided into the footplate grades (i.e. drivers, secondmen and traction trainees and cleaners) and grades other than footplate grades. In the first group, on entry the applicant is required to have acuities of 6/6 in each eye and 6/6 binocularly with the fogging test with correction and also have normal colour vision. The entrants are required to have re-examinations at regular intervals.

In the second group of grades (i.e. other than footplate grades) the following subsections apply.

1 *Class A*. These are required to take tests unaided and must have acuities of 6/12 in each eye and binocularly with a fogging test. If the applicant is wearing a visual correction then he or she must have acuities of at least 6/9 in one eye and 6/12 in the other eye, with binocular acuity of 6/9, again with a fogging test; also the glasses must not exceed ±5.00 D in any meridian. All applicants in this group are required to have normal colour vision. Bifocal lenses are generally permitted but contact lenses are not normally considered suitable. All staff in this group who are likely to use mechanical vehicles or to be on or about the running lines will be subject to re-examination at the age of 40 years and thereafter at 5-yearly intervals.
2 *Class B/clerical staff*. In this group, because of the wide range of employment, the standards laid down are not adhered to so strictly. In general, however, an applicant is required to be able to attain acuity of 6/12 or better in the better eye and at least 6/36 in the poorer eye with or without spectacles. In addition, a near vision acuity of N5 is required. No significant pathological condition may be present.

In general the spectacle correction should not exceed ±5.00 D in any meridian, although this is subject to the discretion of the medical officer.

Definitions of Blindness and Partial Sight

Although this, in terms of registration, does not fall within the scope of the optometrist in practice, a knowledge of the definitions of blindness and partial sight is often useful. An optometrist may not register a patient as blind; this may be carried out only by an ophthalmic medical practitioner or ophthalmologist.

Blindness

The statutory definition for the purpose of registration as a blind person under Section 64 of the National Assistance Act 1948 is that the person is:

> so blind as to be unable to perform any work for which eyesight is essential.

As a consequence of this, two points should be considered:

1 The National Assistance Act 1948 states in the definition 'so blind as to be unable to perform any work ...' and does not relate to a particular occupation or the person's own occupation.
2 It is only the eyesight which is taken into account; any other bodily or mental infirmities are disregarded.

The principal condition to be considered is the visual acuity with correction, either of each eye separately or of both together. As a definition, however, the use of visual acuity alone is not adequate and therefore three classifications of 'blind' exist at present within the meaning of the legislation:

1 *Below 3/60 Snellen acuity:* In general a person whose best visual acuity is below 3/60 may be regarded as blind. Often, however, 1/18 is used as the standard and in this case the person is not considered blind unless there is also considerable restriction of the visual field.
2 *3/60 but below 6/60 Snellen acuity:* A person with visual acuity of 3/60 but less than 6/60 may be considered blind only if this is accompanied by considerable contraction in the field of view. The person is not, however, considered blind within the meaning of the National Assistance Act 1948 if the visual defect is of long standing and is unaccompanied by any material contraction of the field of vision.
3 *6/60 Snellen acuity or better:* A person with 6/60 acuity or better is not normally considered blind. If, however, there is marked contraction of the visual field over the greater part of its extent, and particularly where the contraction appears in the lower part of the field, then the patient may be eligible for registration.

Partial sight

There is no statutory definition of partial sight within the National Assistance Act 1948. The Department of Health and Social Security has advised that a person who is not blind within the meaning of the 1948 Legislation but who is, nevertheless, substantially and permanently handicapped by defective vision whether congenital or through injury or illness does fall within the scope of eligibility for the welfare services which the local authorities are empowered to provide.

The following guidelines are offered when considering whether or not a person should be regarded as partially sighted and when, in the case of a child under 16 years of age, a decision is made as to the type of school recommended.

1 For registration purposes for the provision of welfare services:
   (a) 3/60 to 6/60 with full field
   (b) up to 6/24 with moderate contraction of the field, opacities in the media or aphakia
   (c) 6/18 or better with a gross field defect or marked contraction of the whole visual field.
2 For children when deciding appropriate education:
   (a) severe visual disabilities where education in special schools is required, from 3/60 to 6/24 with correction
   (b) visual impairment where education at ordinary schools is considered suitable if some special consideration is given, better than 6/24 corrected.

The above details should provide a useful background for the most commonly requested vocational requirements. The requirements do, however, vary from time to time and for specific details it may be necessary to contact the relevant governing body.

15

Industrial Eye Protection and the Consumer Protection Act 1987

Safety Regulations

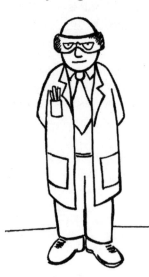

Industrial eye protection plays an increasingly large part in modern optometric practice. Regulations were drawn up in 1974 to replace Section 49 of the Factories Act 1937. The Protection of Eyes Regulations, SI 1974/1681, officially came into force on 10 April 1975. They covered some 35 processes for which approved eye protection were required and five additional situations where persons may be at risk even when not specifically engaged in the particular process.

On 1 January 1993, following an earlier European Directive, the UK Government introduced new legislation on Health and Safety at Work to replace the 1974 regulations. One of the six areas considered within the legislation was personal protective equipment (PPE). The regulations, published under the Health and Safety at Work Act 1974 as Personal Protective Equipment (European Community (EC) Directive) Regulations 1992 SI 1992/3139 cover

- protective aprons and other clothing including garments for adverse weather conditions, gloves, safety footwear, safety helmets and high visibility waistcoats
- equipment such as eye protectors, life jackets, respirators, underwater breathing apparatus and safety harnesses.

The 1993 regulations apply to all workers in the UK with the exception of the crews of sea-going ships.

The publication of these rules led to the revocation of all or parts of existing regulations ranging from The Gut Scraping/Tripe Dressing, etc. Welfare Order 1920 SR&O 1920/1437 to the less evocative Glass Bevelling Welfare Order 1921 SR&O 1921/288 and of more relevance to optometry the complete revocation of The Protection of Eyes Regulations 1974 SI 1974/1681 as amended by SI 1975/303. The regulations relating to eye protection are now taken as the European Normals (EN) standard. A list of these regulations is shown in Table 15.1.

Personal Protective Equipment (EC Directive) Regulations 1992 SI 1992/3139

After the introductory information accompanying these regulations Section 4 relates to the provision of PPE and stresses that provision of such equipment should be considered as the final stage of a safety control system and not just 'an easy option'.

Table 15.1

EN 165 Personal eye protection: Vocabulary
EN 166 Personal eye protection: Specifications
EN 167 Personal eye protection: Optical test methods
EN 168 Personal eye protection: Non-optical test methods
EN 169 Personal eye protection: Filters for welding and related techniques:
  Transmittance requirements and recommended use
EN 170 Personal eye protection: Ultraviolet filters: Transmittance
  requirements and recommended use
EN 171 Personal eye protection: Infrared filters: Transmittance requirements
  and recommended use
EN 172 Sunglare eye protectors for industrial use
EN 207 Filters and eye protectors against laser radiation
EN 208 Eye protectors for adjustment work on lasers and laser systems
EN 379 Welding filters with transmittance variable by time and zone

Under the Management of Health and Safety at Work Regulations 1992 employers are required to identify and assess workplace risk to health and safety and to establish necessary safeguards for employees. When it is considered necessary for protective equipment to be provided for employees it is essential that the equipment is readily available, suitable for the purpose intended and that the employees are trained in the correct use of the equipment. Furthermore where there is a statutory obligation on the employer to supply protective items this must be carried out without charge to the employee.

Any protective equipment purchased for use within the workplace must comply with the relevant legislative requirements. Under the regulations most safety equipment supplied for use at work must be certified by an independent inspection body, which, if the equipment is suitable, issues a certificate of conformity, or CE mark.

Markings for Eye Protectors

The European regulations require that the lenses and the housing of an eye protector must be marked with the relevant information. The markings must be clearly visible on the finished appliance and any markings on the lens must not encroach into the visual area of the device. The characters EN 166 to show the device meets the standard should be clearly marked on the frame or housing but not on the lens. In the case of a one-piece appliance, the complete markings should be applied to the frame only.

Specific symbols are used in lens marking to identify the grade of impact resistance and other specific properties as shown in Table 15.2. The sequencing of the information on the lens is important and should be applied in the order shown in Table 15.3. The filter number relates to the lens filtering properties and may be made up of a shade number prefixed with a designation number indicating the filtering properties against ultraviolet (UV) or infra-red radiation. The designation numbers are shown in Table 15.4. The marking for optical class relates to the optical tolerances to which the lens has been manufactured. The ranges of tolerance are shown in Table 15.5.

Table 15.2   Symbols used in lens marking

Symbol	Property
S	Increased robustness
F	Low energy impact
B	Medium energy impact
A	High energy impact
9	Non-adherence of molten metal and resistance to penetration of hot solids
K	Resistance to damage by fine particles
N	Non-fogging properties

Table 15.3   Sequencing of lens markings

1	Scale number for filter lenses only
2	Manufacturers identification mark
3	Optical class
4	Symbol for mechanical strength
5	Symbol for non-adherence of molten metals and resistance to penetration of hot solids
6	Symbol for resistance to surface damage by fine particles
7	Symbol for resistance to fogging

Table 15.4   Designated numbers for filter markings

2	UV filter and colour recognition may be affected
3	UV filter and good colour recognition
4	Infra-red filter
5	Sunglare filter without infra-red specification
6	Sunglare filter with infra-red specification

Table 15.5   Optical class

Optical class	Sphere and cylinder tolerance	Prism tolerance	
		Horizontal	Vertical
1	$\pm 0.06\,D$	0.75 Out	0.25 Up
		0.25 In	0.25 Down
2	$\pm 0.12\,D$	1.00 Out	0.25 Up
		0.25 In	0.25 Down
3	$+0.12\,D$	1.00 Out	0.25 Up
	$-0.25\,D$	0.25 In	0.25 Down

The result of all this is for lenses of safety eyewear to carry a string of identifiers that enable anyone to determine the characteristics of the lens and the source of the lens. As an example a lens designated to provide medium impact protection, offer resistance to damage from fine particles, having a grade 1 optical class, filtering UV radiation with good colour recognition and shade number 2 manufactured by company X would be marked as:

3-2X1BK

The regulations require that frames or other housings should be marked with the relevant information in a similar way to the marking of lenses. The sequencing of the markings is important and must follow the order as outlined in Table 15.6. The fields of use are shown in Table 15.7 and the symbols for resistance of the material to impact from particles is shown in Table 15.8.

As an example a housing designed for low energy impact and for use where there may be molten metals and hot solids manufactured by X would be marked as:

XEN1669-F

Regulation 5 of the legislation relates to the compatibility of safety items that may be used together. An example would be the use of prescription protective spectacles and a respirator. In the example given only the specified respirator frame would be acceptable. It is the responsibility of the employer to ensure compatibility and that equipment used in combination continues to be effective against the risk or risks defined. If a self-employed

Table 15.6   Sequence of housing markings

2	Manufacturers identification mark
3	The standard number applicable (EN 166)
4	The field of intended use
5	Symbol of resistance to high speed particles

Table 15.7   Symbols indicating field of use for housings

Symbol	Designation
3	Liquids (droplets or splashes)
4	Large dust particles (particle size $>5\,\mu$m)
5	Gas and fine dust particles (particle size $<5\,\mu$m)
8	Short circuit electric arc
9	Molten metals and hot solids

Table 15.8   Symbols indicating resistance to impact from particles

Symbol	Description of impact	Type of protector
-F	Low energy impact	All types
-B	Medium energy impact	Goggles and face shields
-A	High energy impact	Face shields only

person is operating within a risk area it is the responsibility of the individual to ensure that equipment is compatible.

To ensure that protection is adequate Regulation 6 requires the employer or self-employed worker to assess whether the equipment available is suitable for use or not. Such an assessment must include:

- an assessment of any risk or risks to health that have not been avoided by other means
- a definition of the characteristics protective equipment would need to meet the assessed risks
- comparison of the other equipment available with the characteristics required.

This process of assessment would need to be repeated if for any reason it became invalid or if there were significant changes in the working practices or environment.

Regulation 7 relates to the maintenance and replacement of PPE. Once again responsibility is placed on the employer or the self-employed individual to comply. All equipment must be maintained in an efficient state, efficient working order and in good repair. In general equipment should be inspected before being issued and should be further checked by the user before being worn. It should not be worn if found to be defective or if it has not been cleaned.

To assist with good care of safety wear Regulation 8 places a duty on the employer to ensure that appropriate accommodation is available for the PPE when not in use. The storage accommodation provided should be adequate to protect from contamination, loss or damage and in the case of safety spectacles should be a suitable carrying case.

Regulations 9 and 10 relate to training in the use of PPE for employees and information on the responsibility of the individual.

The employer must ensure that employees know:

- the risk or risks for which PPE is provided
- the purpose for which the PPE is to be used and how it is to be used
- the action the employee needs to take to ensure that any PPE provided remains in efficient working order and in good repair.

The employer is again given responsibility for both ensuring the employee understands the training and that the equipment is being used correctly within the working environment. The employee does, however, have an obligation to use equipment supplied in accordance with instruction given and to ensure that it is stored correctly in the appropriate accommodation provided.

A further obligation is placed on the employee by Regulation 11 which requires that any loss of or damage to the safety wear be reported immediately. The reporting process should include arrangements to ensure that the employee does not restart work until the faulty item has been repaired if appropriate or replaced.

The final Regulations 12, 13 and 14 relate to exemptions and changes to existing legislation.

Eye Protection

Eye protection is considered to cover protection against the hazards of impact, splashes from chemicals or molten metal, liquid droplets in the form of chemical mists and sprays, dust, gases, welding arcs, non-ionizing radiation and light from lasers. Protection may be offered as safety spectacles, eye shields, goggles, welding filters, face shields and hoods.

Prescription lenses are available to safety spectacles and some types of protector may be used with standard spectacles and still provide adequate protection. Examples of some of the activities or processes where a risk may occur to the face or eyes and where protectors should be worn are shown in Table 15.9. Protectors should be worn not only by those directly involved in the specific task but also by anyone who may come into contact with the process and be at risk from the hazard.

Categories of eye protector

Safety spectacles: These may include side shields to offer lateral protection, although these should not unnecessarily restrict the field of view, and various levels of lens impact resistance as discussed later in this chapter. Polycarbonate material probably offers the greatest impact resistance for lenses with the lowest weight. Frames can be manufactured in both metal and plastic form with nickel alloys, the most commonly used metal, and polyamide, polycarbonate and cellulose acetate the most common plastic materials.

Eye shields: Similar to safety spectacles these are normally heavier duty and designed with one-piece moulded lenses. Prescriptions cannot normally be incorporated but some are designed for use over standard prescription spectacles.

Safety goggles: More cumbersome generally and less comfortable than spectacles or shields, these normally are of two types:

- cup goggles that have independent lenses and a variable distance between lenses
- box goggles that consist of a flexible plastic frame with one-piece lenses and elastic headband. Many of these can be worn over existing prescription spectacles.

Table 15.9   Examples of activities in which there may be a risk to face and eyes

1	Handling or coming into contact with alkalis, acids and corrosive or irritant substances
2	Working with power tools where chippings are likely to fly or abrasive materials be propelled
3	Working with molten metals or other molten substances
4	Welding operations where intense light or other optical radiation is emitted at levels liable to cause risk or injury
5	Working on any processes using instruments that produce light amplification or radiation
6	Using any gas or vapour under pressure

Goggles can offer all round protection fitting flush to the face and may be ventilated for use in hot conditions. It is important to remember that direct ventilated goggles are unsuitable against the hazards from chemical, gases and dust while indirect ventilated goggles provide unsuitable protection against gas or vapour.

Face shields: Much heavier and bulkier than other forms of protector, these may be hand held or head mounted if fitted with adjustable head harnesses. They protect the face but do not give eye protection against dust, mists or gases. They can be worn over spectacles and are not usually prone to misting. Suitable coatings can be added to the shields to provide protection against heat and other radiation.

Lenses

There are four main types of lens material used in eye protection:

- Glass, a relatively fragile and relatively heavy material, described by the European legislation as mineral. This is not often used for safety wear although it does offer the advantage of good surface durability.
- Toughened glass that is thicker and heavier than normal glass. Toughening may be through chemical or heat process. Surface scratches and abrasions can reduce efficiency and impact resistance and these protectors should be regularly inspected.
- Plastics described in the European legislation as organic material. These have many advantages over glass and are widely used to provide impact resistance. They are lighter in weight and although they are more liable to surface scratching this does not result in reduction in protection although it may affect visibility and therefore efficiency. The three main types of plastic used are polymethyl methacrylate (PMMA), allyl diglycol carbonate (CR39) and polycarbonate.
- Laminated lenses formed by sandwiching a layer of plastic between two layers of glass. They can provide protection by minimizing splintering of the lens material.

Impact resistance requirements

EN 166 provides details of the requirements for different classes of impact resistance that were formerly covered by BS 2092. The EN in addition defines the following five levels relating to impact resistance:

- Minimum robustness – this applies to cover plates and oculars designed to provide a filtering effect but not intended to provide impact resistance. It would be expected that such devices would withstand the impact of a 22 mm steel ball applied at a force of 100 N.
- Increased robustness – for such a classification the unmounted lens has to be able to withstand the impact of a 22 mm diameter steel ball weighing 43 g and striking the lens at a speed of 5.1 m/s. The lens should show no signs of ocular fracture or deformation. The complete eye protector should also be assessed and the requirements relating to increased robustness of complete eye protectors are shown in Table 15.2.

- Low energy impact – the testing of materials for low energy impact require then to withstand the impact of a 22 mm diameter steel ball weighing 43 g and striking the material at a speed of 45 m/s.
- Medium energy impact – this impact resistance is achieved if the material withstands the impact of a 22 mm steel ball weighing 43 g and striking at a speed of 120 m/s.
- High energy impact – to achieve this standard the material must withstand the impact of a steel ball 22 mm in diameter weighing 43 g and striking the material at 190 m/s.

Maintenance of eye protectors

The Personal Equipment at Work Regulations discuss care of protective equipment, etc. and eye protectors should be kept clean as dirty lenses restrict vision that can in turn cause eye fatigue and lead to accidents. In addition lenses that are scratched or pitted must be replaced as they may impair vision or have their protective properties reduced. It should be recommended that eye protectors are issued on a personal basis and are used only by the person to whom they are issued. Following this will ensure that if they are fitted correctly at issue, changes in fit after issue will be minimized.

Good practice guidelines when dealing with eye protection

It should be remembered that by providing protective eyewear as a professional you have undertaken to ensure that the protective eyewear provided is adequate for the purpose. This means that when an industrial order is brought into the practice you spend some time checking that it is able to provide the type of protection needed for the specific processes involved. If you consider that the order would provide equipment that would not adequately offer protection in the working environment then the appliance should not be provided and the company concerned informed.

Ensure record keeping is good. Keep a copy of the original order and specification if from outside. Ensure that the item ordered is suitable for the purpose by asking the patient to outline the conditions in which the equipment is to be used. Record dates of receipt of order, patient examination, dispensing details, order date, date of receipt of spectacles, verification procedure and details of hand-out.

Beware of terminology – never use the terms 'unbreakable' or 'shatterproof' to describe a protective lens or describe a lens as a 'safety lens'. Patients like to hear these terms but no lens can be guaranteed not to break or to shatter under certain conditions.

If any manufacturer warnings accompany products ensure they are passed on to the purchaser and that records show this has been done.

Verification of the finished product prior to hand-out to the patient is very important. In addition to checking lens power check the frame is as ordered, the lenses are free from defects, the lenses fit well into the housing, any tint has been correctly applied and that the lens material is correct.

When issuing a product against a specification ensure it does conform to the required standard and if necessary obtain a written statement of conformity from the manufacturer for your own records.

Where a patient or company is advised of the need for a specific lens material but decides not to follow this advice if you intend to continue supplying obtain a signed statement from the individual/company. The statement should indicate that they have been advised on a material but decided against this advice and selected a lower grade option being aware of the disadvantages.

Consumer Protection Act 1987

This Act received Royal Assent in May 1987 and was in two parts: the first relating to general safety requirements, came into effect in October 1987, and the second relating to product liability, came into effect in March 1988.

Product liability

Before the Consumer Protection Act 1987, anyone injured by a defective product had to prove a manufacturer negligent before they could successfully sue for damages. The Consumer Protection Act removes this need to prove negligence and provides the right to anyone injured by a defective product to sue a supplier without proof of negligence whether or not the product was sold to them.

Action may be taken against the manufacturer of the product, the importer into the EU or, in the case of branding, the supplier who puts their name to the product to give the impression that they are the producers. Other suppliers such as wholesalers and retailers are not liable unless they are unable to identify the producer, importer or 'own brander'. It is not possible to exclude liability under the Act by means of any contract term or other provision.

A defective product in relation to this Act is defined as a product where the safety is not such as persons generally are entitled to expect. Within this a product will not be considered as defective solely because of its poor quality or because a safer version becomes available. A court when reviewing a case would take account of details such as:

1 the manner in which the product is marketed
2 the instruction or warnings given with the product
3 for what the product might reasonably be used
4 when the product was supplied.

For a plaintiff compensation can be claimed for:

1 death
2 personal injury
3 private property valued above a set limit (currently £250).

It must be shown that it is possible that the defect in the product caused the damage.

For the defendant, liability can be avoided if it can be proved that:

- the product was not supplied (e.g. was stolen or counterfeit)
- the state of scientific and technical knowledge at the time of supply was such that a producer of products of the same description as that being investigated would have been unable to discover the defect
- the defect resulted inevitably from complying with the law
- the defect was not present in the product at the time of supply
- the supplier is not in business
- if a producer of components, the defect was due either to the design of the finished product being deficient or to incorrect specifications being given to the component manufacturer by the producer of the finished product.

General safety requirements

This part of the Act makes it a criminal offence to supply unsafe consumer goods in the UK. The Act states that a person shall be guilty of an offence if he supplies consumer goods that are not reasonably safe having regard to all the circumstances. It is this section that is controlled by regulations setting out in detail how specific goods must be constructed and what instructions and warnings must accompany them. These standards will be updated from time to time following approval by the Secretary of State.

This section of the Act differs from product liability in that the general safety requirement applies to anyone who supplies the goods and not just the producer or importer. A 'safe' product is defined in the Act as one that reduces to a minimum the risk of death or personal injury. For the supplier a defence would be to prove that:

1 the goods conform in a relevant respect with an EU obligation
2 the goods conform to any applicable safety standards or regulations approved by the Secretary of State for Trade and Industry for the purpose of the general safety requirement
3 the goods were for export
4 the goods were not supplied as new and were not supplied by way of hire
5 there were no grounds for suspecting that the goods failed to comply with the general safety requirements if supplied in the course of retail business.

Enforcement of the Act is primarily the responsibility of Trading Standards Officers of local authorities, who are given authority to test purchases and limited powers to enter and search premises and obtain information.

In an effort to enable businesses to comply with the requirements, the quality assurance standard for manufacturing procedures BS 5750, was established. The standard set out how companies can establish, document and maintain an effective and economic system for developing and maintaining the quality of their products. All businesses should, however, also ensure that they carry adequate product liability insurance and that records are kept to cover the 10-year potential time scale for product liability claims that would enable identification of the supplier to be made.

Industrial Eye Protection

Key points 1: Categories of eye protector

1 Safety spectacles
2 Eye shields
3 Safety goggles
4 Face shields

Key points 2: Classification of lens impact resistance

1 Minimum robustness (22 mm steel ball applied at a force of 100 N)
2 Increased robustness (22 mm steel ball weighing 43 g striking at a speed of 5.1 m/s)
3 Low energy impact (22 mm steel ball weighing 43 g striking at a speed of 45 m/s)
4 Medium energy impact (22 mm steel ball weighing 43 g striking at a speed of 102 m/s)
5 High energy impact (22 mm steel ball weighing 43 g striking at a speed of 190 m/s)

The Negligent Professional

16

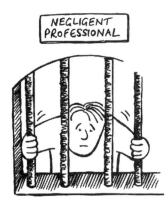

NEGLIGENT
PROFESSIONAL

The law of tort covers many areas but the most common to impact on practice is that of negligence. While many people will have their own concept of negligence in law it has been clearly defined as:

'A breach by the defendant of a legal duty of care which is owed to the plaintiff among others and breach of which causes damage to the plaintiff.'

This may well appear to mirror the type of consideration the General Optical Council (GOC) or the Health Authority (HA) would give to a complaint from a patient. There are however two very big differences – in the civil courts, negligence is proven 'on the balance of probabilities' and not 'beyond reasonable doubt', and if negligence is proven, damages will be awarded to the plaintiff.

The increase in cases coming before the GOC is small compared to the rise in litigation being brought against practitioners for negligence. The College of Optometrists now require evidence of professional indemnity insurance before membership/fellowship can be accepted. Indemnity insurance ensures the patient claim is met. (Insurance is discussed in Chapter 17.)

Is Negligence Easy to Demonstrate?

At face value the definition above seems clear enough and indeed to succeed in an action for negligence the plaintiff is required only to prove the following three conditions:

1 a duty of care is owed personally by the defendant to the plaintiff
2 the duty of care has been broken
3 harm has been suffered as a result of the breach of duty.

As always with the law, however, it is not quite so easy to prove the conditions.

Duty of Care

To prove a duty of care is owed it is necessary to show that a defendant could reasonably have been expected to have seen that a person such as the plaintiff might have been affected by his act or failure to act. The duty of care however can take several forms:

Contractual duty of care

In this situation there should be clear evidence of the duty of care owed, If, for example, an optometrist is registered with an HA to provide sight testing on behalf of the National Health Service (NHS) then when undertaking such tests a clear duty of care has been established. If, however, an optometrist is contracted by an employer to test only the pressure of all the employees and identify any with raised intra-ocular pressure, failure to detect a cataract would not necessarily constitute a breach of duty of care as it did not form part of the contract.

General duty of care

In the case of optometry or dispensing optics if a qualified practitioner sees a patient in practice, that patient would expect the practitioner to carry out any duties with care beyond that expected from an ordinary reasonable person. If a practitioner sets up as a 'specialist' in a particular field such as contact lenses any patient would expect the practitioner to carry out any duties with care beyond that expected from an 'ordinary' optometrist. It is well established in law that a duty of care does exist between the practitioner and patient even though there may be no specific contract or agreement.

The general duty of care however could extend beyond the individual patient seen. For example, a practitioner uses eye drops that reduce a patient's vision but does not warn the patient of the risks of driving. On leaving the practice the patient drives away and is involved in a traffic accident with a third party – the duty of care owed by the practitioner could be seen to extend to the third party.

The logic behind this interpretation is that the practitioner should know that the patient with reduced vision could be dangerous when driving and could therefore foresee the potential for an accident. If, however, the practitioner gives adequate warning to the patient and the patient ignores the advice given, the practitioner could be seen to have completed his duty of care.

Several attempts have been made to define the principle of duty of care and the definition normally quoted is that given by Lord Atkins in Donoghue *v* Stevenson in 1932. It is sometimes called the 'Neighbour principle' and simply says that a duty of care exists when parties are involved in a close and proximate relationship, where one party can reasonably foresee that by his action he is likely to cause harm to the other party.

Breach of Duty

Once it has been established that a duty of care existed between the practitioner and the plaintiff it still has to be proved that the duty of care was broken and that the behaviour of the defendant was sufficiently careless as to make it reasonably foreseeable that some injury to the plaintiff might result.

The courts will expect qualified practitioners to exercise skill and care above that which the courts would expect of an ordinary reasonable person. In assessing whether a practitioner's conduct has fallen below the expected standard the court will look to the opinion of those practitioners of a similar standing. If the practitioner professes a specialist skill (e.g. contact lenses) the standard expected would be higher than for a non-specialist but qualified practitioner.

This is the area where the court in order to determine expectation could use the guidelines issued by the College of Optometrists. The court must be satisfied that the practitioner acts as would an average practitioner of similar standing but the College guidelines specify best practice and not average practice. The College has suggested that 70% of practitioners are complying with the guidelines hence this is the 'normal'. It would be for the court to listen to arguments and then decide on whether the College guidelines represented an average view. As the professions elected body and in the absence of any other guidelines the court may take the view that they are representative of what a patient might realistically expect.

The issue of experience is also relevant here. It has been determined that should a newly qualified practitioner undertake a procedure the practitioner will be judged on the same standards as an experienced practitioner performing the same procedure – no allowance is made for lack of training. In this way the duty is 'tailored to the act not the actor'. To avoid liability it would require evidence that the novice recognized his lack of experience and sought the advice of a more experienced colleague.

A court will not automatically consider a practitioner liable if a diagnosis is incorrect. What is expected is that due care and skill has gone into arriving at the decision. It is therefore important to understand when further diagnostic tests are necessary and when referral to a specialist is the most suitable option.

Harm has been Suffered

As stated earlier duty of care, breach of duty and harm arising must be proven for action on negligence to succeed. It does not matter how careless a course of action may be, if no harm results there is no liability.

The breach of duty may not need to be the sole contributory factor to the harm resulting but must have materially contributed. The general rule for the standard of proof in all civil cases is 'but for the defendant's fault, on the balance of probabilities, the injury complained of would not have occurred'. In essence this means the plaintiff has to persuade the court that there was a greater than 50% chance that the action of the defendant resulted in harm.

Let us look at the example of a patient attending for examination with a small retinal detachment. A cursory examination is carried out and the detachment is not noted. The following day the detachment increases and the patient attends a casualty unit and is treated so that no permanent damage results. In this case it is likely that detecting the detachment one day earlier would have made little difference to the outcome and negligence may be hard to prove. If however the patient assumes that all is well after the visit to the optometrist and does not attend the casualty but continues for 2 weeks before seeking a further opinion it could be very different. The detachment is enlarged and reaching the macula area and re-attachment now becomes difficult resulting in permanent damage to the retina. In this case the original practitioner would be liable for negligence.

Damages

'Damages' is the financial measure of the harm suffered. When considering a case the court will attempt to ensure that the injured party is maintained in the position that they would have been had the harm not occurred. Normally consideration will be given to two aspects the first relating to matters leading up to the case reaching court, for example, loss of earnings, special equipment purchases, medical expenses, etc. and the second dealing with future financial loss. The first is relatively easy to determine the second is not.

When considering the future the court will try to put a figure to:

1 Compensation for pain and suffering resulting from the harm.
2 Affect on enjoyment of life.
3 Future loss of earnings.
4 Loss of earnings capacity and prospects.
5 Loss of benefits such as pension.
6 Future expenses including medical care.

Period of Action

It can often take some time before the results of a particular action or failed action become apparent and, while mindful of this, the law is also aware of the strain of waiting. In order to provide an equitable solution the law provides a time frame within which action may be taken. There is a limit of 3 years starting either from the date on which the action occurred or the date on which harm as a result of the action became apparent. It is possible for a court to allow action beyond this period but the circumstances would need to be exceptional.

In the case of a minor there is a further variation and the 3-year period commences from their eighteenth birthday when they attain majority.

Protection from Claims

It is not possible for complete protection from the possibility of a claim for negligence being brought. To minimize the risk a practitioner can either:

1 Carry out every test on every patient and ensure that all the minor variations in results are accountable.
2 Refer every patient with even the most minor of problems.
3 Play Russian roulette and take the view that 'it will never happen to me'.
4 Complete a thorough routine using tests to investigate symptoms and observations of the patient and to support results found during examination.

The first three options are not sustainable in a real practice situation leaving the fourth one as the only realistic mode of practice.

It is for this reason that insurance is necessary to cover the risk of a claim occurring. In some cases the amounts awarded in damages can run to seven figures enough to affect most optometrists if they had to raise the funds themselves! The issue of indemnity insurance will be addressed in Chapter 17.

Key points 1: For negligence to be proven

1 It must be shown that a duty of care existed
2 The duty of care must have been breached
3 Harm must have resulted from the breach of duty of care

Key points 2: Courts will look to see that

1 Due care and attention were given
2 Further diagnostic tests were carried out where necessary
3 Any referral made was at a suitable point in time

The Need for Insurance

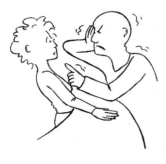

In Chapter 16 the implications of civil action were discussed with particular reference to negligence claims. To protect yourself as an optometrist and to ensure financial support for any damages due to a patient succeeding in an action it is normal to take out some form of insurance. Insurance cannot alter the decision of a court or a professional body but it can provide the finances to fight a case where insurers deem it appropriate and also provide a sum to cover the cost of damages awarded.

As the frequency of litigation increases and the value of damages awarded increases, the cost of insurance is likely to increase. However, competition is fierce within the insurance industry and often as premiums rise the range of benefits offered is also improved.

Who Needs Professional Insurance?

Any qualified member of the profession should have a form of professional liability insurance. The Health Act 1999 provided the Secretary of State for Health with an enabling power to introduce a law requiring all professionals to have liability cover. If you are in practice and come into contact with members of the population in general you are at risk of action being taken for negligence. As set out in the chapter on negligence even the most careful of practitioners can err or misjudge.

What Type of Insurance Should I Have?

In the case of professional liability it is sensible to take out insurance covering four main aspects:

1 *Professional liability cover:* This is legal liability cover in respect of advice given for a fee. It should be noted however that if you act as an expert witness you may need to increase the level of and/or modify the terms of your policy to ensure adequate cover.

Claims made under this cover are rare in optometry tending to relate to bodily injury of one sort or another. To illustrate the point no claims have been made to date in respect of this cover within the Federation of Opthalmic and Dispensing Opticians (FODO) insurance scheme.

2 *Products liability cover:* This is legal liability that can arise from accidental injuries sustained by or accidental loss of or damage to the property of a third party arising from defects in goods sold or supplied or from the repair, servicing, cleaning or alteration of goods.

An example of a claim made under this aspect would be for injury caused following a screw falling out of spectacles. The vast majority of patients survive such episodes in tact but there is a risk of damage here.

3 *Third party liability cover:* This may be defined as legal liability arising out of premises risks only.

A claim made by a patient who had walked into an unsigned glass door within a practice and been injured would be an example of this type of claim.

4 *Public liability including medical malpractice:* This cover relates to legal liability for third party bodily injury or disease and is by far the most common type of insurance claim made by optometrists.

Examples of claims falling within this category range from missed pathology to damage following the provision of incorrect contact lens solutions.

It is also necessary to ensure that your policy includes cover for legal defence costs. Most policies of this nature would include the costs involved in defending an action brought by the individual concerned.

If you are involved in special activities such as shared care schemes it is worth talking to your insurance adviser about the costs of additional cover for these specialized situations that may fall outside the scope of normal optometric cover. While standard malpractice insurance should cover you for most eventualities any treatment being carried out (e.g. the use of therapeutics) may not be automatically included.

Where you act as an expert witness as mentioned earlier it may be that your standard professional liability insurance cover will need to be upgraded. In addition to an ophthalmic malpractice cover it may be necessary to take out a separate professional indemnity insurance.

What Happens if I Stop Work?

It is possible to take out two forms of professional liability insurance. The first is based on 'occurrence' such that the insurer 'on risk' at the time of the incident deals with the claim irrespective of when the claim is made. The second is based on 'claims made' under which a claim is dealt with by the insurer that is 'on risk' at the time the claim is made. The advantage of the 'occurrence' format is that you are covered even after you decide to stop practising. In the case of 'claims made' policies you would need to take out what is called run off cover.

There is a further complication when you switch from 'claims made' to 'occurrence' format. You would be well advised to take out retrospective cover for the years leading up to the change. Most insurance advisers will be pleased to discuss these issues with you and it is essential that you are clear in your own mind exactly which form of insurance you have.

How Much Cover Should I Take Out?

This is obviously up to the individual but currently the College of Optometrists expect their members to have a level of cover of at least £1 million and the FODO cover is for £2 million.

When an individual is injured, and liability for the accident is found to lie with another party, the subsequent court case determines the amount of money in damages they receive to compensate for their loss. This loss relates to earnings and expenses and can extend to cover the rest of their life. Taken into account are age, life expectancy and the level of earnings received currently.

Often Insurance Companies will attempt to come to an agreement without the case going to court. For many practitioners who consider themselves to be at no fault this can be extremely disconcerting. The fact that a case is settled by agreement without admission of liability is however a way of reducing potential costs and reducing the time scale over which the particular case may spread. This should reduce the inevitable pressure that builds on all those involved. This course of action is taken when a successful defence action is not possible, for example, due to poor record keeping.

Previous claims settled range from sums of a few hundred pounds covering costs and professional fees for solicitors to £100,000 to provide an out of court settlement. As patients become more aware of their rights and the role of the practitioner as a detector of pathology is more accepted it is likely that the number of claims will continue to rise and the level of settlement may increase.

How Great a Risk is There?

The simple answer to this is too great a risk not to take out insurance cover. The number of cases each year may be small in terms of the total number of patients seen but if you are the practitioner involved it can be devastating. The practitioner has to contend with the worry, the fall in confidence, the potential knock-on effect with other patients and the effect on family members. More than this there is also the time taken to finalize the case (sometimes it can take years before a resolution is agreed) and the time involved in meetings and preparing information.

It is unlikely that the total number of claims to insurers made by the optical profession is accurately known. On the basis of figures through the FODO insurance system in the 2 years to September 2000 less than 1 in 50,000 eye examinations results in an insurance claim each year (FODO update). That still means approximately three cases for each practitioner during their lifetime! This low number is not so surprising as minor disagreements and complaints will be sorted within the practice and only more serious cases will reach the insurer.

Types of Complaint

An analysis of the complaints dealt with by FODOs insurers (AON Risk Services) over a 2-year period provides the following basic breakdown of areas involved:

Failure to detect	33%
Incorrect prescription causing problems	32%
Wrong contact lens solution	7%
Contact lens related damage	9%

NCT problems	4%
Spectacle breakage while wearing	7%
Incorrect diagnoses	3%
Service and property related	3%
Other	2%

Within the failure to detect category the following conditions are the most commonly cited:

Glaucoma	25%
Cataract	14%
Retinal detachment	19%
Brain tumour	15%
ARMD and CSR	5%

It can be seen that there is a wide variation in the cause of complaints and underlying pathologies.

An incorrect prescription sounds an innocent and simple enough error to deal with but it is the consequences of the error that cause difficulty. Many claims are made after a patient has had a fall causing injury that may be attributable to the incorrect spectacles. Alternatively claims are made where a patient is involved in a car accident and cites the incorrect prescription as a potential cause. Almost 30% of claims involving an incorrect prescription have such added spice! In some ways this type of complaint should be the easiest one to eliminate by increasing the checks made on spectacles progressing through a practice.

How Do I Get Insured?

For those individuals working for members of FODO, insurance cover is provided for work undertaken on behalf of the employer and for Association of Optometrists (AOP) members individual insurance can be taken out through the AOP Services. Similarly Association of British Dispensing Opticians (ABDO) provide an insurance service to its members. If, however, you do not wish to be part of these schemes there are underwriting insurance companies that regularly advertise in the professional journals who will tailor insurance to your particular needs. Whoever provides your insurance should supply you with a detailed schedule of the cover provided and any exclusions – check this very carefully and make sure it meets your specific needs.

Remember that insurance cover is only provided for risk notified to the insurer and if you practice techniques which are not considered 'normal' practice or you provide services from premises not notified to the insurer you may invalidate any claim. The insurer is there to help and any queries will normally be dealt with professionally and effectively.

The College of Optometry insists on a signed statement indicating that adequate insurance provision has been arranged as a requirement for continued membership. If you are unsure of your position check with your employer or with your insurance provider – it is not worth the risk of being uninsured or underinsured.

Key points 1: Insurance cover for optometrists should include

1 Professional liability
2 Products liability
3 Third party liability
4 Public liability including medical malpractice

Key points 2: The majority of claims by optometrists and dispensing opticians are for

1 Failure to detect/refer a pathology or abnormality
2 Problems caused by providing an incorrect prescription
3 Contact lens related damage
4 Incorrect contact lens solutions provided
5 Spectacle breakage causing damage

18

The European Union and European Legislation Affecting Optometry

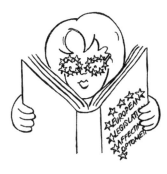

The professions of optometry, ophthalmology, dispensing optics and optical mechanics are interwoven into a complex structure throughout Europe. Each member country of the community has its own established hierarchy, protected titles and definitions. In terms of professional status, freedom and academic training the optometry profession in the UK has always been seen as ahead of the equivalent professional groups in the other member countries.

The situation has been, and continues to be, changing with improvements in training and professional legislation throughout Europe and the opening up of the supply of spectacles by the unqualified and removal of the National Health Service (NHS) right to examination for some groups in the UK. While the UK may still be ahead, the gap between the profession here and the professions in Europe is slowly shrinking.

The UK entered the then European Economic Community in 1972. Since that time negotiations have been taking place between the various optical bodies in the member countries and European officials in an attempt to produce legislation acceptable to all parties and which allows freedom of movement between countries for qualified optometrists. The negotiations on behalf of the UK profession have been carried out through the Joint Optical Consultative Committee on the Common Market. As the health services offered and the form of funding vary widely throughout Europe it is little wonder that progress has been slow.

More recently the commission for optical and optometric organizations in the European Community (EC) (GOMAC) has become more active and helped member states to understand better each other's needs and difficulties. In addition the European Council of Optometry and Optics (ECOO) has put substantial effort into developing optometry in Europe. ECOO is the confederation of the leading professional bodies representing optometrists and opticians in 23 countries in Europe including all the member states of the European Union (EU).

The situation is very much in a state of flux and many countries have optometrists in practice due to custom and practise even though they are not recognized by legislation and a 'blind eye' is turned to their activities by regulators.

General Directive on the Mutual Recognition of Higher Education Diplomas

This document (89/48/EEC), intended to harmonize professional groups within the member countries of the EU, has laid down the basis for optometric interchange within Europe. The Directive is extremely general in its coverage and does not require prior harmonization of education and training. In order to produce equivalence it is understood that the optometrist in each state covered by the proposal will complete a full course of upper secondary education followed by successful completion of a 3-year full-time course leading to a higher education diploma. The Directive also covers those who take an equivalent 3-year full-time course on a part-time basis.

Because of the differing national legislation throughout the community, experience and knowledge of varying areas of clinical optometry may be restricted in certain individuals. The legislation, again by its general nature, does not interfere with this but provides for training and qualification of optometrists intending to migrate to be assessed to identify any significant shortfalls. Once identified it is for the migrating optometrist to overcome these differences by further training, supervised practice or examination as determined by the accepting country. The optometrist will always be allowed to return to the home country however and would carry the extended qualification.

There was inevitably a scramble of activity before the introduction of this Directive with many European countries now boasting a new 3-year full-time university course in optometry. This will obviously enable member states to participate in the movement of qualified personnel. In addition, AESCO (the Association of European Schools and Colleges of Optometry) has been discussing the development of a syllabus and examination structure for the introduction of a European Diploma in Optometry. This, combined with a slow but steady movement of individuals between countries, could see the expansion of optometry and harmonization of the profession in Europe. Initial examinations have been held but the poor uptake and outcomes have led to a review of the structure of the syllabus and the whole examination process.

In order to understand the magnitude of the effect that harmonization will have it is interesting to review briefly the state of the optometric profession in some EU countries.

Belgium

Two organizations exist in Belgium, each supporting an optometry course. The older established and most supported organization is L'Association Professionelle des Opticiens de Belgique; the other more recently established is the Union Nationale des Optometristes et Opticiens de Belgique. Upon successful completion of a sponsored course a candidate is offered a diploma: 'd'opticien/optometriste', signed by the Minister of Health. The Diploma falls within the 'Cours Techniques Secondaires Superieurs' classification and legally entitles the recipient to use the title 'opticien/optometriste'.

A royal decree of 1964 ensured the continuation of the privilege of objective and subjective refraction and contact lens fitting by the opticiens/optometristes. A further development, by a decree in 1975, was the recognition of a two-tier profession by the introduction of a separate branch of dispensing opticians in addition to opticiens/optometristes. The law, however, recognizes members of the profession as opticians and not as optometrists although their role covers many of the functions normally carried out by optometrists elsewhere. In Belgium as well as objective and subjective refraction the members of the profession are able to refer to medical practitioners but are not allowed to use diagnostic instrumentation.

Denmark

The optometric or ophthalmic profession in Denmark is relatively new although it carries out 90% of primary eye examinations. It was established as a profession, separate from the crafts of instrument making and watch making, by a government decree in 1954. Two organizations exist in Denmark to represent optometrists, and a third represents both ophthalmologists and optometrists. The groups are the Danish Society of Opticians, the Danish Society of Optometry and the Danish Contact Lens Association (the last representing the two professions).

Following lengthy negotiations and legislation there is statutory registration of optometrists in Denmark. Optometrists are allowed to carry out objective and subjective refraction, use diagnostic instruments, refer to medical practitioners and fit contact lenses following further training. There are some restrictions applied but despite this the Danish optometrists have established the right to receive payment for certain categories of service within the national health programme. There is no university course available, the training being via colleges of technology and this may cause problems for harmonization.

France

The basic qualification for optometric registration in France at the present time is the 'Brevet de Technicien Superieur Opticien Lunetier'. Despite some 5500 people holding this qualification, ECOO has estimated that 90% of eye examinations are carried out by ophthalmologists. The legal attitude of the French Courts to optometry was established by a ruling made in 1927, which stated that it was an illegal practice of medicine for an optician to attempt to direct a wearer of spectacles to use a particular prescription found by the optician.

Registration and licensing of optometrists was established in 1944. The original bill laying down the terms for registration made it illegal to fit spectacles to children under the age of 16 years without a medical prescription, to use objective methods for determining the refraction and to use an ophthalmoscope. After the original bill the restrictions hardened rather than eased. The year 1958 saw the introduction of a regulation making it compulsory for the majority of French citizens to take out health insurance which required an ophthalmologist's authorization for reimbursement of refraction and spectacle charges. In 1962 a stipulation appeared in the Journal Officiel de La Republique Francaise stating:

> The manipulation of instruments used in the determination of the ocular refraction are medical acts ... to be carried out only in accordance with Article L.372 (1~) of the public health law.

The restrictions have not stopped there, and the practice of orthoptics was denied by decree between 1965 and 1970. There is now, however, a move towards better training and qualification standards, which may be the turning point for the French optometric profession.

University courses have been offered in Paris and Marseilles and this has resulted in optometrists now holding an optometric licence following a 4-year university diploma course. The combination of the harmonization directive from the EU, professional group pressure and the establishment of university courses should see France on course for rapid change in optometry.

Germany

Two basic divisions exist in the optometric profession in Germany: the 'Augenoptikermeister' or master optometrist, and the 'Augenoptiker' or state examined optometrist. The Augenoptikermeister is the better placed of the two, having full privileges to:

- own or manage a practice or business
- sell and fit prescription eyewear
- undertake visual examinations for the purposes of prescribing spectacles
- fit and sell contact lenses
- fit and sell low vision aids
- receive reimbursement for services and materials from health insurance offices
- provide training for optical apprentices and assistants.

A series of court cases has established that under German legislation the acts of refraction, both subjective and objective, should not be considered medical acts and more recently that the use of a non-contact tonometer and the assessment of peripheral vision are acceptable. Other aspects of optometric practice such as orthoptics are not undertaken except in co-operation with an ophthalmologist. There is no legislation to cover the referral of patients where ocular pathology is detected although this does happen. In order to practise a government license is required. It is still the case that ophthalmologists carry out the majority of eye examinations.

One difficulty on the road to harmonization is that the profession in Germany does not call itself optometry and has no direct comparison in the UK. In the same way they do not call themselves dispensing opticians and this is likely to add to the confusion.

Unification meant that the East German situation had to be evaluated. Reports suggested that the Master of Optometry diploma awarded after successful completion of a technical college course of 2 years' duration allowed refracting for insurance purposes. It seems that integration of the two systems has not been a major difficulty.

Greece

It is probably unfortunate for the optometric profession that just before completion of EU membership formalities in 1979 the Greek government passed a bill making it illegal to practise optometry in Greece. All eye examinations are carried out by ophthalmologists, and optometrists may only dispense.

The present situation is likely to remain for the foreseeable future although negotiations have taken place between members of the professional groups in other European countries and representatives of the Greek Ministry of Health and Welfare. The talks covered legislation, training, scope of practice and the benefits of optometric service. It is to be hoped that this will lead to a more tangible change in optometric legislation.

Ireland

The situation of ophthalmic optics in the Republic of Ireland is very similar to that in the UK. There is a two-tier system of ophthalmic and dispensing opticians who are regulated and registered by the Opticians Board established by the 1956 Opticians Act. In fact the Opticians Board has a function very similar to that of the General Optical Council (GOC) in the UK, being responsible for training standards, registration and the introduction of regulations. A form of health insurance exists under which free eye examinations are provided and a range of spectacles is offered free of charge and optometrists carry out 90% of primary eye examinations. A 3-year full-time course is available at Dublin College of Technology.

Italy

Registration in Italy as an 'ottico' (plural, 'ottici'; ottica optics) is available via courses at several institutions. Further advanced courses at a number of the institutions, leads to an optometric diploma. In addition to these existing courses, legislation through the Italian Chamber of Deputies led to the establishment of university schools of optometry. It is perhaps this that has produced the current position for optometry in Italy.

Optometry existed in Italy without statutory regulations until 1928. The enactment of law No. 1264 on 23 June 1927 regulating disciplines auxiliary to the health profession was followed by a royal decree issued on 31 May 1928 which defined the duties and privileges of ottici. Article 12 of the decree restricted the refracting rights of the ottici by requiring the authorization of a medical physician when selling spectacles and lenses to the public. There were exceptions to the general rule, including simple myopia, presbyopia and duplication of spectacles, for all of which the ottici could prescribe.

The government definition of the scope of ottici stipulated the need to know objective and subjective refraction and visual analysis techniques as well as assessing eyewear in terms of the medical prescriptions available and the fitting of contact lenses upon medical authorization. This broad definition gave considerable force to the proposal that the ottici were overqualified to act simply as 'dispensing opticians'. Optometry is still however limited in its scope of practice.

Although the tendency still seems to be for the ophthalmologists to carry out the eye examinations, the situation is changing. The area of contact lenses is also of interest in Italy. A 1972 decree by the Ministry of Health prevented ophthalmologists from selling contact lenses. This has led to an estimated 90% of all contact lens fitting being carried out by ottici.

Luxembourg

The training to qualify as an independent optician in Luxembourg is long: following an apprenticeship with a practising optician and success at examination there follows a period of practical education in opticians' workshops and theoretical education. On completion of training the student takes final exams to qualify as a master optician which gives the right to practise as an independent optician and carry out objective and subjective examinations, use diagnostic instruments, fit contact lenses and supply spectacles. No university courses are available in Luxembourg where there are only a small number of optometrists' practices. Overseas qualifications are, however, acceptable for registration as a master optician. To practise an optometrist is required to be licensed by the Ministry and by the professional body.

Netherlands

Optometrists in Holland enjoyed relative freedom as regards eye examinations until the revision of the Medical Practice Act in 1938. In this Act, however, a definition of ophthalmology made it clear that the optometrist would be permitted to carry out only subjective examination. The statute laid down that the use of trial lenses and a letter chart was not a medical act in law, but that examination of an organ and advice as to correction or alleviation of defects was. The Dutch profession accepted that this meant that retinoscopy and ophthalmoscopy were illegal acts.

A step forward from this position towards the recovery of professional status came with the establishment of formal registers of opticians as laid down by royal decree in 1966. This led to a commission report which included recommendations that a specific law be enacted to authorize optometrists to work in the areas of opticianry, optometry and contact lens fitting.

The introduction in 1988 of a 4-year university course in optometry offered at the University of Utrecht provided the impetus for change.

Section 34 of the Individual Health Care Professions Act 1998 has finally allowed for the regulation of Optometry as a profession in its own right. Section 5 of Order of Council 297 laid down on 4 July 2000 defines the scope of practice of an optometrist and importantly allows for the use of pharmaceutical agents to aid in screening for disease. The title of optometrist is also protected under the legislation and may only be used by those practitioners who have graduated in Optometry. Refraction and dispensing of optical aids are covered elsewhere in the new Act and are not exclusive to optometry.

Portugal

At present the optometric profession is attempting to promote the profession via its university courses. There is no legislation restricting practice in Portugal and the majority of practices are dispensing with a limited number of optometrists. The professional organization is the Uniao Profissional dos Opticos e Optometristas requires optometrist to be licensed and they have through the 4-year registrable university degree course managed to promote optometry. Optometrists do carry out objective and subjective refraction and refer to medical practitioners and it is likely that this status will be formalized by regulation in the near future.

Spain

Developments here in which ophthalmologists are involved in the teaching of pathology within the university optometry course should allow optometrists to provide NHS examinations. The existing 3-year course is likely to be expanded to 4 years to allow for development of the course.

All optometrists are registered with the Colegio Nacional and only optometrists are allowed to sell and supply spectacles. Optometrists carry out subjective and objective refraction, use diagnostic instrumentation and refer to medical practitioners.

European Recognition of Qualifications

The European Directive on Mutual Recognition of Professions, effective from 4 January 1991, has as mentioned earlier provided further impetus for the development of optometry in Europe. The university course (or equivalent) is now becoming the normal in most countries and it is hoped that formal recognition and registration could follow. While there is still confusion among the member states as to definitions and equivalence for syllabi the situation is improving steadily.

Optometry appears in the EU (Recognition of Professional Qualifications) (Amendment) Regulations 2000 (SI 2000/No.1960) as a 'Profession regulated by law or public authority'. It is listed in Schedule 1 Part 1 and the designated authority is the GOC. Interestingly dispensing opticians are listed in Schedule 2 Part 1.

The place of optometry in the UK as the goal that others were striving for may not however remain for too long. The hunger among the other EU countries to improve their profession is contrasted against the UK government's moves in the past 10 years to dismantle the NHS and at one stage consider deregulating the profession. This has changed somewhat more recently and the advent of co-management programmes has meant that UK optometry is playing an increasing role in the provision of eye care. However with the remainder of Europe improving steadily the UK is no longer as far ahead as previously thought.

19

Computers in Optometric Practice and the Data Protection Act

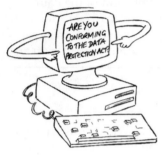

In the late 1980s there was a sudden explosion in the number of software houses providing programs for computerization of optometric practices. Aggressive marketing by computer firms linked with the optometrist's shrinking market at that time following changes in the NHS legislation led to a sudden awareness among practitioners of how they thought computerization could improve their business. Slowly the software companies merged or fell by the wayside and while computerization is here to stay, the whole basis on which it is viewed is changing.

How then, does the average optometrist in practice set about deciding on whether a computer system would be useful, and if so which system to choose? The first step must be a thorough review of the routines within the practice with particular regard to whether they would lend themselves to computerization. The routines normally quoted as suitable are reminders and stock information, both of which are easy to computerize. Additional areas that may be looked at are, for example, supplier's lists, solutions and sundries files, dispensing information, finance and eventually patient records. If existing manual systems are operating smoothly and efficiently, and to your own requirements, then computerization may be a luxury that is not needed. However, computerization can give you access to a wealth of information, and you need to ask whether that information would be of value if it were available to you.

Options for Computerization

Available optical practice management programs

These are software alternatives that have been specifically geared to the needs of a practice; they should have been tried and tested (always ask how many users and how long since the first and still operating system was installed), and therefore most of the irritating bugs removed. The disadvantage is often that they offer far more than the individual optometrist would want, simply because they are a compilation of the needs of a half dozen pioneer practices. They do allow you to contact existing users (ask for a list – there may be someone you know operating the system) and find out all the information and problems that the salesman will not necessarily give.

Adapt an existing off-the-shelf database or business program

This option is for those with a real interest in computing and plenty of free time. It does, however, allow you to design exactly what you feel you want within the constraints of the database, and is considerably cheaper than a customized optical package. You do not, however, get the back-up or the contact with other professionals using a similar system or identical system, and when you have problems you are on your own.

Pay a computer consultant to design you a system

Optics by its nature is a mixture of retailing, business management, clinical information, technical information and accounting. It is sometimes difficult for someone with no expertize to understand the link – on the other hand, it is sometimes refreshing to have an outsider to review your systems. If you decide on this option you will need to hammer out exactly what you require in some detail with whoever is invited to prepare software and you will then need to revise it once a system is operating. This option could be very expensive and time consuming, and in the end leave you with a system that meets none of your needs adequately but does a bit of everything and it is not the option for the computer naive.

Points to Remember

Plan carefully and start slowly

Inevitably, despite the best laid of plans, you will find that once you have installed and run the system it is not quite what you wanted. Until you have a system available you do not know what you need! The system must be flexible and you must be prepared to adapt routines as well as the system.

Start with only what you need to computerize

The computer salesman will tell you that they can computerize everything – and they probably can – but for most individual practices there may be only certain functions that benefit from computerization, for example, payroll, reminders and sundry stock. Be ready to start with the basics and work up to full computerization when the bugs have been ironed out. Do not get carried away by the 'glitz' of it all. Try to look at systems that will build together should you find computerization ideal and need to expand.

Consider alternatives

There are numerous management services firms who will subcontract computerization requirements, for example, reminder letters. It may be worth investigating the cost and the time saving of this alternative. Additionally, if you are only using the system for reminders study your existing manual system and investigate the time that could be saved, if any, before deciding on computerization.

Be sure of what you want and expect to pay to get it!

Once you have decided that computerization is for you and you know which areas you wish to computerize and what information you wish to store and retrieve, discuss this with an expert. Do not choose the cheapest system without ensuring that it can do all that you want it to speedily and with room for memory expansion should you decide to add to your requirements. It may be an asset to have a system that you can modify yourself if you have computer literacy and therefore, one that has a reasonable language. In addition, if you choose hardware that is readily available, compatible with most software, proven, and flexible, you will be able to use the system for other business packages should you so decide or even for games when children come to be examined.

Always stay in control

The specialist computer adviser is there as the role suggests, to advise and do not, therefore, be 'steam rollered' into something that does not apparently give an advantage even if the adviser waxes lyrical. Always check the costs of everything – telephone links may be exciting, but would a fax be cheaper for what you really need? Do not use what you do not need, even if an option is available on the software you are running.

Ensure back-up

At the end of the decision-making and installation, you are going to need someone who is prepared to train you effectively and to be available to answer queries as they arise. Make sure that whoever provides the software is prepared to take on this trouble shooting role and make sure that whoever supplies the hardware is prepared to sort out problems quickly. You will find that by locking yourself into a reputable company you will also be updated as new advanced versions of the software become available. Ensure however, that the updates are an improvement for your particular needs, always bearing in mind that if you do not take the update you could end up as the only user of a particular version and, therefore, not able to obtain support back-up.

Check the software manual

Any system that has been operating for some time should have a corresponding manual available. This may be your salvation in times of stress when the help line is engaged and everything seems to have crashed. It should be intelligible, well indexed, comprehensive and up to date.

Mistakes

1 Do not expect the computer to solve all the organizational problems of a practice. If anything, the computer will create organizational difficulties in a disorganized office. Always remember that the computer is only as good as the information that is fed into it – if you fail to keep the information up to date your whole system can fall around you.
2 Do not expect the software to slip neatly into the practice. It may be too simple, it may be too complex – the staff may be unwilling or unable to cooperate with the installation and ongoing use. Remember that the system that you install should be flexible but so should the routines within the practice and aim for a 'best fit' situation.
3 A computer system is not static. Software is constantly being upgraded

and enhanced and the practice has to be prepared to adapt to the changes if it wants technical support maintained.

4 An essential requirement for any system is software and hardware back-up. Do not assume that a system has no problems and that you do not, therefore, need support.

5 Do not assume that a computer system already does a particular job simply because it is the commonest routine in your existing manual system. You may be doing something that no one else has thought of.

6 Do not feel that because a system works manually it must work better when computerized. There is no logical reason to transfer the appointment diary to computer. Both for ease of view and for changing information a pencil, diary and eraser are far simpler.

7 If you employ people in the practice who are going to need to use the system, do not think that they necessarily share your enthusiasm and commitment to the project. Also, do not think that by sitting them in front of a computer screen and leaving them they will suddenly be able to operate the system. You will need to arrange training and by involving staff in system selection you could improve motivation.

8 Computerization is not automatically a way of saving staff costs. In fact, it is often more expensive to computerize but the theory is that by making everyone more efficient you make more money and you offer a better service to your patients.

9 Do not put off the computer routines for another day. Ensure that enough time is allowed to complete the day's entries on the actual day, otherwise the system will become out of date and information will be forgotten.

10 Even if the system appears to be running smoothly, take a regular back-up of the data – normally daily, but certainly weekly – any longer and if the system crashes it may take months to sort out data.

It is impossible to decide the best system for all in a section of this type, as there are so many individual considerations. Hopefully, the points made here will be used as a guide when investigating the options available and when running any system that you install. Computers can be fun, but they can also be the cause of nightmares when they are not running in the way that they should. As with everything else in optics, confidence is of paramount importance so ensure that you have confidence in the system, the company, the support and your ability to use the system.

Data Protection Act's of 1984 and 1998

The increasing use of computers to hold personal data led to the introduction of the Data Protection Act in 1984. The Act gave new rights to people to enable them to view information about themselves, challenge it if appropriate, and in certain circumstances, claim compensation. The order was enacted for health records as SI 1987/1093 Data Protection (Subject Access Modification) (Health) Order in November 1987.

This Statutory Instrument allows access to data held on computer for

1 the person directly involved (data subject)
2 a person authorized by the data subject

3 a person authorized to act on behalf of the data subject

4 a person having a power of attorney.

On making a written request and payment of a fee, any of the above may be supplied with a copy of any personal data held about a data subject. Any such request must be responded to within 40 days and failure to do so entitles the applicant to complain to the Data Protection Registrar (this title changes to Data Protection Commissioner in the 1998 Act). The information may be supplied as a print-out, written text or typed and should have any accompanying explanations that are required to understand the information.

In the case of health care records held on computer SI 1987/1093 allowed for modified access to data where it was considered that disclosure was likely to cause serious harm to the physical or mental health of the data subject or another person. Restrictions were also imposed where disclosure of data could lead to identification of another individual other than a health professional involved in the health of the patient.

If in any doubt about the legal standing of an individual in relation to receipt of information then it would be sensible to seek legal advice or to contact the Data Protection Commissioner to seek advice.

A register of data users complying with the 1984 Act (and it is a criminal offence not to be registered if the exemptions are not met) is held by the Data Protection Commissioner's Office. The entry in the Register contains the data user's name and address together with:

1 Description of the personal details which the data user holds.

2 Outline of the purposes for which the data are to be used.

3 Data sources.

4 To whom the data may be disclosed.

5 Any overseas countries or territories to which the data user may wish to transfer the data.

The Commissioner can refuse registration should the information given prove inadequate but once registered the data user commits a criminal offence if they knowingly:

1 Hold personal data not described in the Register entry.

2 Hold or use personal data for purposes other than described in the Register entry.

3 Obtain personal data or information to be placed in personal data from a source not described in the Register entry.

4 Disclose personal data to a person not described in the Register entry unless covered by a non-disclosure exemption.

5 Transfer personal data to an overseas country or territory not described in the Register entry.

The introduction of the 1998 Act extended the protection to non-electronic-based forms of data storage. It also overhauled the Access to Health Records Act 1990, but made little difference to the rights of patients to access their health records. Clinical records in practice would be treated as sensitive personal data under the terms of the Act. Where the data processing and storage is in manual form there appears to be no need to register although this is still under review and the regulations relating to access still apply even if an individual is not registered under the terms of the Act. If however electronic data processing is involved the regulations to register are as before.

One change is the view of the Data Protection Commissioner that implied consent to process information may not be acceptable. This would mean that you would need to seek implicit consent from a patient to a record of the consultation being kept. TYhis is in conflict with the professional bodies' recommendations to maintain detailed and accurate records of all patient visits and it could be that an exemption is made during the clarification process.

All data processed for medical purposes must be kept confidential. This means that the patients consent should be sought before information is passed to another health professional or third party. The Data Protection Commissioner has provided the view that information relating to dispensing of an appliance may be passed on with the verbal consent of the patient. Any information relating to the clinical notes of the patient should only be passed on with the written consent of the patient. At present there are different interpretations of whether a refractive result constitutes dispensing or clinical data.

The transfer of data does not extend to the purchase of record cards as this is considered within the terms of the Act as a change in ownership and not publication of information.

A further complication in transfer of patient data is created by the Caldicott report on handling patient information. Health Authorities and Trusts have appointed 'Caldicott Guardians' who have responsibility for ensuring the maintenance of good practice when handling patient data. The principles involved are currently unenforceable but as contracts in the future are likely to be more rigorous it is likely that evidence of confidentiality of patient information will be required.

Any optometrist keeping patient records or other personal details on computer should be registered with the Data Protection Commissioner. It is possible that in the future holders of manual data on patients will need to register and this should be monitored. If in any doubt or should further information be needed details can be obtained from Data Protection Commissioner, Wycliffe House, Water Lane, Wilmslow, Cheshire, SK9 5AF, UK; Tel: (01625) 545700.

Key points 1: Access to data held on computer is allowed for

1 The person directly involved (data subject)
2 A person authorized by the data subject
3 A person authorized to act on behalf of the data subject
4 A person having a power of attorney

Key points 2: When using computerized record systems the following details must be registerd with the data protection commissioner's office

1 Name and address of data user
2 Description of personal details to be held
3 Outline of purpose for which data are to be used
4 Data sources
5 To whom the data may be disclosed
6 Any overseas countries to which data may be transferred

20

Aspects of General Law Relating to Optometric Practice

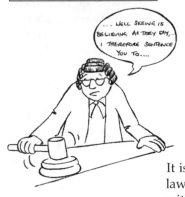

It is important for a practitioner to be aware of certain aspects of general law that apply to everyday situations. Some of these aspects are associated with familiar daily routines such as contract law relating to a practitioner contract with the Health Authority (HA). It is important that other areas, for example, partnership and sale of goods, are understood as they are again likely to affect professional life. Some of the more commonly met legislation will be outlined below. If ever a problem arises, however, it is important that the advice of a qualified solicitor is sought.

Partnership Law

The law on partnership is based on the Partnership Act 1890, with special provisions for limited partnership dealt with in the Limited Partnerships Act 1907. According to the 1890 Partnership Act:

> Partnership is the relation which subsists between persons carrying on business in common with a view of profit.

The rights and duties of the partners among themselves will vary in accordance with the partnership agreement, but there are a number of statutory requirements within the Partnership Act 1890 that will be presumed to apply wherever an agreement is lacking in detail. These requirements are:

1 partners are each entitled to share equally in both the capital and the profits of the firm, but do not have any rights to payment for working on partnership business
2 disputes relating to the operation of the firm are settled by a majority decision, except in cases where unanimity is called for, such as the introduction of new partners or the change of business of the firm
3 unless specific arrangements are made for sleeping partners, every member of the partnership has the right to participate in the management of the firm
4 partners have the authority to inspect the books relating to the partnership business at any time, and books should be kept at the place of business of the partnership for this purpose
5 members of the partnership have a right to be indemnified by the firm for liabilities incurred in the course of executing the firm's business.

The Partnership Act 1890 laid down certain provisions covering the formation of a partnership:

1 No partnership may be formed consisting of more than 20 persons except for banking where the permitted number is 10, according to the Companies Act 1985. Solicitors, accountants, auctioneers, estate agents and members of the stock exchange are also exempted under the Companies Act 1967 and the Board of Trade Regulations 1968.
2 If partners intend to carry on business under a name which is not the names of all the partners, such a name must be registered together with the names of the partners, and a certificate of registration obtained (Registration of Business Names Act 1916).
3 A partner cannot compete directly with the firm he belongs to, nor derive personal benefit from the firm's business, without the prior consent of the other partners.
4 Each partner in a firm is treated as an agent for the firm, and his fellow partners are legally liable upon contracts made or torts committed by a partner while acting on the firm's behalf.
5 Partners are jointly liable on the firm's contracts and jointly and severally liable for the firm's torts to the last penny of their personal fortune unless the partnership is a limited partnership formed and registered under the Limited Partnerships Act 1907. A limited partnership must still have at least one general partner whose liability is unlimited; if, however, a limited partner participates in the management of the firm then the limitation of liability is lost.

When forming a partnership it should be treated as a business arrangement and should therefore be put on a strictly business footing. Agreements should be drawn up by a solicitor, and, although the terms of any such agreement will vary considerably, the following items should be included:

1 *The duration of the partnership* (this may be for a fixed number of years or for an indefinite period).
2 *Shares in capital and profits*. The agreement should specify the share of the capital and the share of the profit to which each partner is entitled. Provision may be made for a gradual increase in share holding for a junior partner working his way into the firm.
3 *Provision for retirement*. An agreement should specify in detail the procedure for the retirement of partners and will usually give the continuing partners the right to acquire the outgoing partner's share on specified terms including the payment of a lump sum and/or an annuity to the outgoing partner. Such details should also apply in the case of the death of a partner.
4 *Competition*. A clause may be introduced to prevent a partner who leaves the firm from carrying on a business in competition with the partnership within a specified distance.
5 *Expulsion*. The agreement should specify the circumstances under which a partner may be expelled or forced to retire from the firm.
6 *Arbitration*. As no agreement covers all eventualities, however carefully it is planned, it is possible to maintain a clause that provides for arbitration by an independent body in cases of dispute within the partnership.

Any partnership, however formed, may be dissolved under the following circumstances:

- By the expiry of the period of agreement.
- By the completion of the particular undertaking for which the partnership was formed.
- By the death or bankruptcy of any partner where no arrangements for this circumstance have been included in the partnership agreement.
- By the mutual agreement of the partners.
- By order of the court following an application made by any partner under the following circumstances:
  - (a) where a partner is suffering from a mental disorder or is otherwise incapable of carrying out his obligations to the firm
  - (b) where an allegation is made that a partner's conduct is liable to prejudice the successful continuance of the business or that his behaviour is in breach of the partnership agreement, making continued co-operation almost impossible
  - (c) where a partnership in commercial practice cannot make a profit
  - (d) where the termination of a firm is seen to be a fair and equitable solution to the firm's problems.

Corporations/Companies

Before 1844 most industrial and trading business was carried on either through partnerships or unincorporated associations. After that date, however, various Companies Acts were laid down culminating in the Companies Act 1948, the Companies Act 1967 and the Companies Act 1985. The result was that businesses were given the benefit of incorporation, particularly the benefit of limitation of liability of their members. Registration of a company is effected by depositing the following documents with the Registrar of Companies:

1 *Memorandum of Association.* This is the company charter, defining its constitution and the scope of its power. If the company is limited by shares then the memorandum must state:
  - (a) the name of the company with 'limited' as the last word in the name
  - (b) the country in which the registered office will be sited
  - (c) the objects of the company
  - (d) a declaration that the liability of the members of the company is limited
  - (e) the amount of share capital to be issued and the type of share.
2 *Articles of Association.* These are regulations governing the internal management of the company. They define the duties of the directors and the mode or form in which the business will be carried out.

There are three types of registered company defined in terms of the level of liability:

1 A registered company limited by shares in which the liability of the members to pay the debts of the company is limited to the amount unpaid on their shares, if any.

2 A registered company limited by guarantee in which the liability of members to pay the debts of the company is limited to the amount guaranteed and payable only if the company is wound up.
3 An unlimited company in which the liability of the members to pay the debts of the company is unlimited.

Registered companies may also be divided into two classes based not on the limit of liability but according to the number of members, as follows:

1 *Public companies*. These have a minimum of seven members and have shares which are freely transferable on the share market.
2 *Private companies*. These have a minimum of one member and a maximum of 50 (not counting members who are past employees) and shares which are not freely transferable on the open market. The articles of association of such companies generally contain some provision for the sale of members' shares.

In law there are advantages and disadvantages to incorporation. The more important legal consequences of incorporation are:

- the corporation or company can be sued in its own name and may be prosecuted for criminal offences; it may also sue under its own name
- once incorporated the company forms a legal personality separate from the personalities of its members whom it can therefore sue and who can sue the company, and with whom the company can make contracts
- the corporation can, within the limits of its powers, trade like an ordinary individual
- the corporation or company can make contracts in its own name through human agents
- the corporation can own and dispose of property like any ordinary individual.

When a corporation has been created by law then it must act within the powers that have been granted; this is the so-called *ultra vires* doctrine. The powers of a corporation are defined in the memorandum of association of a registered company. Any contract made outside the powers of the company according to the *ultra vires* doctrine will be considered void.

Once formed, there are specific legal means for the termination of a company. The agreement may be terminated:

1 By the Registrar of Companies striking the company name from the register, having first satisfied himself that it is no longer trading.
2 By voluntary winding up after mutual agreement of the members of the company.
3 By compulsory winding up following an order of a court due to
   (a) inability to pay debts
   (b) failure to commence business within 1 year of formation
   (c) failure to hold the statutory meeting or to file the statutory report or to maintain minimum numbers.

Contracts

A contract is a legally binding agreement, i.e. one that will be enforced by the courts. According to Sir William Anson, a contract may be defined as:

> A legally binding agreement made between two or more persons, by which rights are acquired by one or more to acts or forebearances on the part of the other or others.

In practice, contracts form a basic part of the business and clinical activities of the practitioner. Certain essential factors are required for a simple contract to be considered valid in law. An agreement will be enforced, therefore, only when the following elements exist:

1 *Offer and acceptance.* There must be an offer made by one party and this offer must be accepted by the other party.
2 *Intention.* There must be an intention to create legal relations between the parties concerned.
3 *Capacity of the parties.* Each party involved must have the legal capacity to make the contract.
4 *Consent must be genuine.* A contract will not be considered valid if consent has been obtained by fraud or duress, for example.
5 *Consideration must be present*; i.e. some right, interest, profit or benefit.
6 *Legality of objects.* The objects and aims of the contract must be within the law.
7 *Possibility of performance.* The contract must be one which is capable of being performed.

All of the above elements are required to be present for a simple contract to be considered legally binding. If one or more is absent from the contract then one of the following may be considered:

1 *Contract void.* In this case it is destitute of legal effects; i.e. it is not a contract and no legal rights may be conferred on the parties concerned.
2 *Contract voidable.* In this case the contract may be made void at the instance of one of the involved parties.
3 *Contract unenforceable.* Here the contract would be valid but is not enforceable because of:
   (a) the absence of evidence of the contract
   (b) the absence of the legally required format.

The simple contract is not the only type of contract that exists in law, but it does tend to be the most important and by far the most common type. For information regarding other forms of contract, it is advisable to consult a solicitor.

Law of Tort

A branch of civil law that is of importance to the optometrist is the law of tort. This may be defined as:

> A civil wrong for which the remedy is a common law action for unliquidated damages and which is not exclusively the breach of a contract or the breach of a trust and other merely equitable obligation.

As the definition states, tort is a civil law term; originating in France, it means simply 'a wrong'. It is used in English law to denote wrongs committed by one citizen against another serious enough to merit the award of compensation to the injured person but not serious enough to amount to a breach of criminal law.

Frequently contract law and law of tort overlap, although certain distinctions can be made. The following points are therefore of importance:

1 If the plaintiff cannot sue without proving the existence of a contract then the action is for breach of contract and not for tort.
2 In contract law the duties of the parties concerned are fixed, usually by the same parties, whereas in law of tort the duties are fixed by the law.
3 A person who is not a party to a contract cannot sue for breach of contract even though the breach may have caused that person damage. If, however, a defendant's action is also a breach of a legal duty then any person affected can sue in tort.

The most common form of present day action for tort is in the tort of negligence (see Chapter 16). To succeed in an action for negligence the plaintiff is required, for all practical purposes, to prove the following:

1 There exists a duty of care owed personally by the defendant to the plaintiff.
2 The duty of care has been broken.
3 Harm has been suffered as a result of the breach of duty.

Tort of negligence may then be defined as:

> A breach by the defendant of a legal duty of care which is owed to the plaintiff among others and breach of which causes damage to the plaintiff.

To prove condition 1, above, requires that the defendant could reasonably have been expected to foresee that a person, such as the plaintiff, might be affected by his act or failure to act. This is not always easy to prove.

If the court agrees that a duty of care was owed then the plaintiff still has to prove that the duty was broken and that the behaviour of the defendant was sufficiently careless as to make it reasonably foreseeable that some injury to the plaintiff might result. Even if the defendant is able to show that he exercised care to the best of his ability, this may still not be considered adequate by the court. It seems that the courts tend to take the stand that a reasonable man takes extra precautions where the chances of an accident are greater or where the consequences of an accident may be more serious.

At this stage the plaintiff still has the task of proving that damage has resulted from the negligence committed and that this damage is a direct result of the incident.

It is possible for an act of negligence to lead to action both for breach of contract and for tort. For example, if A privately hires an optometrist, O, to carry out a sight test on a bedridden relative, B, and as a result of the examination, O negligently causes harm or fails to detect an abnormality in B, then two possible courses of action are available:

1 A may sue O for breach of a contractual duty of care.
2 B may sue O for the tort of negligence, i.e. the breach of the legal duty of care.

Sale of Goods Act 1979, the Sale and Supply of Goods Act 1994 and the Supply of Goods and Services Act 1982

With the recent legislative changes to 'open up competition' the business side of the optometric profession has come to the fore. One very important area of the general law associated with this side of ophthalmic practice is covered by the Sale of Goods Act 1979 and the Sale and Supply of Goods Act 1994. These acts consolidate the existing legislation including Sale of Goods Act 1893 and Supply Goods (Implied Terms) Act 1973. This legislation however only applied to the sale of goods and to assist a buyer of services by providing similar protection the 'Supply of Goods and Services Act 1982' was introduced.

The following conditions and warranties are implied in every contract for the sale of goods unless they are expressly excluded by the parties:

1 A condition that the seller has or will have a legal right to sell the goods at the time the transaction is to occur.
2 A condition in sales by sample that the bulk will correspond to the samples on which an order was based. In addition, the buyer should be given ample opportunity to compare sample and bulk, and the goods must be reasonably free of any defect not likely to be apparent on such examination.
3 A condition that in a sale where the seller provides goods as described by the buyer, the goods will correspond with the description.
4 A condition or warranty of quality or fitness for any purpose is implied only in the following circumstances:
   (a) where the seller is a specialist dealer in the goods sold and the purchaser makes it clear that he relies on the seller's judgement, a condition is implied that the goods shall be reasonably fit for the purpose intended if the purpose is specified
   (b) where the seller is a dealer in the goods sold, there is an implicit condition that they shall be of merchandisable quality (i.e. of a generally acceptable quality)
   (c) an implied warranty or condition may be incorporated by the custom of a particular trade
   (d) an express warranty or condition does not negate a condition or warranty implied by the Sale of Goods Act 1893 unless it is inconsistent therewith, in which case the express term excludes the implied term;
   (e) a warranty that the buyer shall enjoy quiet possession
   (f) a warranty that the goods shall be free of any undisclosed charges or encumbrances in favour of any third party.

In the law of contract, where there is the possibility of misrepresentation the maxim has always been *caveat emptor* or 'let the buyer beware' and this still applies to private sales. The Sale of Goods Act applies only to sales made in the course of a business. It is essential in the sale of goods that the buyer does everything possible to protect himself/herself. Protection should be in the form of obtaining as much information and as many assurances as possible from the seller.

Trade Descriptions Act 1968 and 1972

Further Acts of Parliament relating to the sale and supply of goods is the Trade Descriptions Acts 1968 and 1972. These are Criminal Law Acts that attempt to improve the accuracy of traders in describing the goods and services they offer to the public; it, too, is particularly relevant to the optometric profession following the recent changes in the legislation. The relationships between the Trade Descriptions Act 1968, the Sale of Goods Act 1893, the Misrepresentation Act 1967 and contract law can be very complex. The main point, however, is that the consequence of breaking the Trade Descriptions Act is a criminal prosecution. This means that under the Acts the outcome of any action is punishment and not just rescission of a contract or payment of damages.

The basic offences created under the Trade Descriptions Act 1968 are:

1 applying a false trade description to goods
2 supplying goods to which a false trade description has been applied.

It is possible to adapt these general rules to cover services as well as goods. There will be no offence committed if:

1 the inaccuracy is considered trifling
2 the seller can show that the goods were believed to be as described and with reasonable care it was not possible to show that the goods differed from the description
3 all reasonable precautions were taken and it can be shown that the misdescription was the result of a genuine mistake, the fault of someone else or due to a cause beyond the control of the defendant.

The Trade Descriptions Act 1968 details the points which may be found to constitute a trade description. These include:

- the composition of the goods
- the method of manufacture
- the quantity
- the size
- the fitness for a specific purpose
- the performance in test and general use
- the date or place of manufacture
- the identity of the manufacturer
- the previous ownership of the goods
- statements that the price has been reduced or is lower than the recommended price.

Prosecutions under this act are brought by a local authority, usually following an enquiry by the Trading Standards officials. Proceedings may be instituted on their own initiative or following a complaint from a member of the public. This legislation is also applicable to the unregistered seller of spectacles.

Shops Act 1950 and Shops (Early Closing Days) Act 1965

These Acts of Parliament relate to staff hours, trading days and times, and aspects of staff working conditions. The details of requirements under these acts will vary from area to area due to local council exemption orders and it is therefore advisable to seek local advice regarding details.

Fire Precautions Act 1971 and Fire Precautions (Non-Certificated Factory, Office, Shop and Railway Premises) Regulations 1976

These Acts and regulations are concerned with the protection of people in the event of fire. Under these regulations:

- there must be reasonable means of escape in the event of fire
- there must be suitable equipment for fighting the type of fire likely to occur
- the equipment should be maintained in efficient working order
- all fire exits must be conspicuously marked.

The regulations relating to fire are very important, and a fire certificate is required for premises other than those where:

- 20 or fewer people are working at any one time
- 10 or fewer persons are employed to work at any one time elsewhere than on the ground floor
- there are other factory, office or shop premises in the same building but the sum total of employees is 20 or less.

In most areas the local fire prevention officer is willing to help with advice and information and should be consulted if in doubt about requirements.

Workplace (Health Safety and Welfare) Regulations 1992

These regulations resulting from a European Union (EU) directive were aimed at tidying disparate sets of regulation such as parts of the Factories Act 1961 and the Offices, Shops and Railway Premises Act 1963. They set general requirements in four main areas:

- working environment, for example, temperature, ventilation, lighting
- safety, for example, windows, passageways, floors
- facilities, for example, toilets, rest area, clothing storage, drinking water
- housekeeping, for example, maintenance of equipment, cleanliness.

Health and Safety at Work Act 1974

This Act applies to all persons at work, however small the business, including the self-employed, but excluding domestic servants in private households. It is designed to protect the people at work and the health and safety of the general public who may be affected by the work environment. According to the act, it is the duty of every employer to ensure, as far as is reasonably practicable, the health and safety of employees. In addition to providing and maintaining a safe working environment the employer has to provide information, instruction, training and supervision reasonably to ensure the health and safety of employees. An adequate first-aid kit also must be provided and a first aider available (Health and Safety at Work (First Aid) Regulations 1981).

Under the legislation, the employee has a duty to conform to statutory requirements, to take reasonable care to avoid injury and not to misuse or interfere with equipment provided. Where five or more employees are working, a written statement must be prepared outlining general policy with regard to health and safety at work and a safety officer should be appointed. The details should be displayed in the form of a notice or be available within the work premises SI 1989/682.

An employer under the terms of the Control of Substances Hazardous to Health Regulations 1994 (COSHH) has to assess the risks arising from the use of hazardous substances. This would cover methylated spirits or acetone, for example, that may be used within a practice environment. Once assessed, steps need to be put in place to warn employees of the risks identified. Harmful micro-organisms and other biological agents are also included within this legislation and therefore the problems of sterilization of trial contact lenses or other items likely to be contaminated by vCJD, for example, would be covered.

Although the Health and Safety at Work Regulations are designed to protect employees in the workplace there is also a duty of care owed to all visitors to the premises. This would include, for example, patients, sales representatives and the window cleaner. This duty is also covered within the Occupiers Liability Act 1957.

Disability Discrimination Act 1995

Section 21 of this Act lays down requirements to make goods, facilities and services more accessible to disabled people. The regulations required service providers to work to a timetable:

- From October 1999 change policies, procedures or practices that make it impossible or difficult for disabled people to use a service; overcome physical barriers by providing a service by a reasonable alternative method.
- From 2004 take all reasonable steps to remove, alter or provide means of avoiding physical features that make it unreasonable difficult or impossible for disabled people to use a service.
- From 2001 all new premises to ensure no physical barriers to prevent a disabled person accessing services.

The European Union Directive on Visual Display Screen Equipment and Its Implications for UK Optometry

The EU issued on 29 May 1990 Directive 90/270/EEC which required all member states to implement the proposals within the Directive between 1992 and 1996. The title of the document was 'Council Directive on the Minimum Safety and Health Requirements for Work with Display Screen Equipment' and was the fifth individual Directive on the introduction of measures to encourage improvements in the safety and health of workers at work.

The increasing numbers of office and industrial environments using visual display units (VDUs) meant that this particular directive had far reaching consequences to very large numbers of people within the community. By its nature the directive was binding on member countries and the Health and Safety Executive (HSE) in the UK prepared a discussion document before making recommendations to the Secretary of State for a legal framework.

Regulations were introduced into the UK under the Health and Safety (Display Screen Equipment, (DSE)) Regulations 1992 SI 1992/2792. The regulations were wide-ranging and covered:

- analysis of the workstation
- requirements of the workstation
- daily work routines of users
- eyes and eyesight
- provision of training
- provision of information
- exemption certificates
- extension of regulations outside Britain.

Although an optometrist involved in provision of a DSE service needs to be familiar with all the aspects involved it is the eye and eyesight section that is of particular interest. The HSE produced guidance to assist in interpretation of the regulations that proved very useful.

Within the terms on eyes and eyesight an employer is required to ensure that an eye and eyesight test is provided to any employees who are defined as users. The tests must be carried out by a competent person and provided at regular intervals determined by the clinician. There should be no charge to the employee for this service.

An appropriate eye and eyesight test has been defined by the HSE guidance as being one as defined by the Opticians Act 1989. Where screening is made available it does not negate the rights of an employee to request a full eye and eyesight test.

Where it is determined that an employee requires a corrective vision appliance for use solely on the DSE then the employer must make arrangements to provide this at no cost to the employee. Should the employee use the appliance for other work or decide to choose an appliance that is different to the range offered by the employer there is no liability on the employer to make a contribution towards the cost.

Employer/Employee Legislation

Contracts of employment

The Employment Protection (Consolidation) Act 1978, as amended by subsequent legislation, requires that all employers provide, within 2 months of the commencement of employment, written particulars of certain fundamental terms of the contract of employment. The following terms must be included in the written statement:

1 The name of the employer and of the employee.
2 The job title, which should include a short description of the scope of work intended.
3 The date of commencement of employment.
4 The scale of remuneration and the intervals of pay.
5 The normal hours of work (any expected overtime commitments should also be recorded).
6 Holiday entitlement and rates of holiday pay, including public holidays.
7 Particulars of any pension scheme or pension and whether the employee is contracted out of the state pension scheme. If no pension or scheme is available, this must be noted.
8 Terms and conditions relating to incapacity due to injury or sickness. If there are no such details then the contract need not say so.
9 The period of notice an employee is required to give and is entitled to receive.
10 Details of previous employment if counting towards the period of continuous employment.
11 Disciplinary rules and procedures.
12 Details of the person, by name or job description, to whom the employee can go in the case of any grievance, together with details of the grievance procedure.

Exemption from the above requirements is an employee whose spouse is the employer.

The Part-Time Workers (Prevention of Less Favourable Treatment) Regulations 2000 ensures that part time or temporary staff are offered benefits such as holiday entitlement on a pro-rata basis.

Equal Pay Act 1970

The Equal Pay Act 1970 (as amended by the Sex Discrimination Act 1975) and the Sex Discrimination Act 1975 were introduced in order to remove discrimination against women in employment. These acts are inter-linked with Article 119 of the Treaty of Rome and subsequent directives.

The Equal Pay Act is concerned with:

1 instances where an employee of any age of one sex receives less favourable rates of pay than an employee of the opposite sex under a contract of employment with the same or an associated employer
2 instances where an employee of any age receives less favourable contractual terms than an employee of the opposite sex.

The provisons are that in both cases the work they are doing is:

1 the same
2 broadly similar such that any differences are not of practical importance
3 of equal value as determined by a 'job evaluation'.

Sex Discrimination Act 1975

This act complements the Equal Pay Act 1970. It established the Equal Opportunities Commission to investigate and eliminate wherever possible discrimination of all types in employment. Under the terms of the Sex Discrimination Act 1975, it is unlawful for an employer in Great Britain to discriminate against a man or a woman on the grounds of his or her sex or marital status. The legislation covers recruitment, terms and conditions of employment, training schemes, promotion, benefits and facilities. Only employers with five or more employees (whether full time or part time) are liable under the terms of the Sex Discrimination Act 1975.

Rights of the employee on dismissal

There are three ways in which dismissal can occur in normal working circumstances, according to the Employment Protection (Consolidation) Act 1978:

1 The employer can terminate the employment either verbally or in writing.
2 A contract may have been for a fixed term and come to an end without being renewed.
3 The employer may be in breach of a fundamental term of the contract of employment, entitling the employee to leave without notice. (This particular case is called 'constructive dismissal'.)

If an employer dismisses or is found to have 'constructively dismissed' an employee, the dismissal may be considered unfair unless it was for one or more of the following permissible reasons:

1 Related to the capability or qualifications of the employee for the type of work for which he was employed.
2 Related to the employee's conduct.
3 A redundancy situation existed.
4 A statutory restriction was placed on the employer or employee such that continuation of the employment contravened the law.
5 Some other substantial reason.

The provisions for unfair dismissal do not apply in the following situations:

1 where an employee has not completed 52 weeks of continuous reckonable service
2 where the employee is part time, normally working fewer than 16 h/week
3 where the employee has reached retirement age

4 where the employee is on a 1-year fixed contract and has agreed in writing during that time to forgo any right to compensation at its expiry
5 in certain lock-out or strike situations
6 where the total length of employment does not exceed 2 years and during that period there have been not more than a total of 20 employees, provided that employment commenced on or after 1 October 1980
7 where the employee is the employer's spouse.

In addition to the above general circumstances, there is a set procedure that must be followed in cases of dismissal to prevent the case being considered unfair by virtue of default in procedure. The guidelines are contained in a government-produced Code of Practice that is regularly updated. At present the following recommendations should be complied with:

1 All employees should receive copies of the employer's disciplinary procedure(s).
2 Employees should be entitled to answer any complaints against them and be accompanied at such a meeting by a colleague or union representative.
3 No employee should be automatically dismissed for a first offence unless it involves gross misconduct.
4 The case should be fully investigated before any action is taken and responsibility for action should not rest with the immediate superior but with a higher authority.
5 A full explanation of any penalty and its reasons should be given to an employee, together with notification of the right to appeal and the procedure to be followed.
6 Where disciplinary action other than dismissal is contemplated, this should be preceded by a formal warning in the case of minor offences and a written warning for serious offences.
7 A criminal offence committed outside of the employment should not be considered an automatic reason for dismissal.

The whole area of unfair dismissal is a complicated one, changes rapidly, and the above simply outlines some of the details. For further information it is advisable to consult a solicitor who has specialist knowledge of industrial law.

Redundancy

Parliament first introduced the idea of redundancy payments as compensation for staff being made unemployed due to specific reasons. Basically, any employee is eligible for redundancy payment, with the following exceptions:

1 where the employee has not completed at least 2 years of continuous service since the age of 18
2 where a man is 65 years or over or a woman is 60 years or over
3 where the employee is a part-time worker generally employed for fewer than 6 h/week
4 under the conditions of certain fixed-term contracts
5 the employee is the employer's spouse

6 where an employee refuses an offer of suitable alternative employment within 4 weeks of the redundancy date.

The term 'redundancy' is meant to cover termination of employment attributable wholly, or in the main, to:

1 an employer ceasing or intending to cease the business upon which the employee was working
2 an employer ceasing or intending to cease the business at the place at which the employee was working
3 requirements of the business changing such that the particular kind of work of the employee is no longer needed or is needed less or is likely to be needed less.

The employer is not liable for the whole of any sum paid as redundancy pay and may, under the terms of the Employment Protection (Consolidation) Act 1978, claim a rebate on the payment from the Redundancy Fund using the relevant form obtained from the local Department of Employment Office.

Employer's Liability (Compulsory Insurance) Act 1969

In order to protect employees this law required that all employers insure against personal liability for personal injury to their employees. To comply with the act employers must:

1 take out an approved policy with an authorized insurer against liability for bodily injury or disease resulting from and during the course of employment
2 display a copy of the certificate of insurance in an easily accessible position where employees are able to view the certificate.

This is a selection of the law that affects optometrists in their business environment. As the law is constantly changing and open to interpretation anything stated in the above is only to be considered as correct at the time of publication. Should the optometrist ever become caught up in a legal dispute it is essential that proper legal advice be sought.

Appendix 1
National Health Service Forms

GOS 1   Application for NHS sight test

Fill in Part 1 and sign and date Part 2. If you are under 16 or incapable of signing, your parent, carer or other person responsible for you should sign.

Part 1   Patient's details

*delete as appropriate

Mr/Mrs/Miss/Ms*:   Previous surname:

Other names: Date of birth: /   /

Address:

Postcode:

#if known

Date of last NHS sight test: /   /   NHS no#:   N.I.no#:

Tick any box which applies to you

☑ I am 60 or over   ☑ I am under 16†

☑ I am a full time student aged 16, 17 or 18† and attend:

†You may be entitled to an optical voucher if you are in one of these groups. Ask the person who tests your sight.

School/College/University*:

Address:

Postcode:

I/my* partner receive(s):

☑ Income Support†   ☑ Income-based Jobseeker's Allowance†

☑ Working Families' Tax Credit†   ☑ Disabled Person's Tax Credit†
   (maximum rate *or* reduced by £70 or less)   (maximum rate *or* reduced by £70 or less)

Person getting the benefit/Credit* if not the patient:

Name: Date of birth: /   /

☑ I/my* partner have HC2 certificate number:

☑ I am registered blind/partially sighted* with the Local Authority below

☑ I suffer from diabetes/glaucoma* – my GP's details are below

☑ I am considered to be at risk of glaucoma by an ophthalmologist at the hospital below

☑ I am 40 or over and am the parent/brother/sister/child*of a person who has or had glaucoma

☑ I have been prescribed complex lenses under the NHS optical voucher scheme

Optician's use only
Evidence not seen

GP/Local Authority/hospital*:

Address:

Postcode:

☑ I have had a sight test at home because I cannot leave home unaccompanied

Part 2   Patient's declaration

This is my application for an NHS sight test. I declare that the information given on this form is correct and complete and I understand that if it is not, appropriate action may be taken. I confirm proper entitlement to an NHS sight test and for the purpose of checking this, I consent to the disclosure of relevant information, including to and by the Inland Revenue and Local Authorities.

I am:

** If you are incapable of signing, your parent, carer or other person responsible for you should sign and give their name

☑ the patient   Signature**:   Date: /   /

☑ the patient's carer or guardian.   Signature**:   Date: /   /

Name: *(in block capitals)*

Address: *(if different from above)*

Postcode:

NOV. 00

GOS 1

Part 3 Practitioner's declaration

✓ I have tested the sight of the person named on this form on *(date)* / /

✓ I have made a domiciliary visit to conduct this sight test to one patient at the address in Part 1

✓ I have made a domiciliary visit to several patients at the address in Part 1

This patient was the:

✓ 1st patient at that address

✓ 2nd patient at that address

✓ 3rd or subsequent patient at that address

This patient was unable to attend the practice for their sight test because:

✓ The patient was referred to their GP

✓ A prescription showing no change or statement was issued

✓ A new or changed prescription was issued

✓ A voucher was issued:

Type: Supplements: ✓ *Complex* ✓ *Prism* ✓ *Tint*

CLAIM I claim:

✓	the current NHS sight test fee	£
✓	the domiciliary visiting fee for:	
✓	1st patient at the address in Part 1	£
✓	2nd patient at this address	£
✓	3rd or subsequent patient at this address	£
	Total of claim for sight test	£

Note: *In the case of a re-test at less than the standard interval, please specify appropriate reason.*

Address where sight test took place: *(in capitals/stamp)*

Address *(if different)* where payment should be sent: *(in capitals/stamp)*

I declare that the information given on this form is correct and complete and I understand that if it is not, action may be taken against me. For the purpose of verification of this claim, I consent to the disclosure of relevant information. I claim payment of fees due to me for work carried out under the NHS optical voucher scheme.

Practitioner's signature:

Practitioner's name: *(in capitals/stamp)*

Date: / /

Ophthalmic list number:

GOS 2 Patient's optical prescription or statement

If you need new glasses or contact lenses, give this prescription to the optician when you order them. A prescription may be valid for up to two years, so keep this form safe.

Part 1 Patient's details

* delete as appropriate

Mr/Mrs/Miss/Ms*:	Previous surname:
Other names:	Date of birth: / /
Address:	
	Postcode:

 # if known

Date of previous NHS sight test: /   /   NHS no#:   N.I.no#: ☐☐☐☐

Part 2 Prescription or statement

I tested the sight of the above patient today in accordance with the regulations and:

Tick the box to show what action was taken

- ☑ The patient was referred to their GP
- ☑ A prescription showing no change *or* a statement was issued
- ☑ A new or changed prescription was issued
- ☑ A voucher was issued:

Type: ☐   Supplements: ☑ *Complex*   ☑ *Prism*   ☑ *Tint*

R I G H T	Sph	Cyl	Axis	Prism	Base		Sph	Cyl	Axis	Prism	Base	L E F T
						Distance						
						Near						

Comments:

I declare that the information given on this form is correct and complete and I understand that if it is not, action may be taken against me.

Practitioner's signature:	Practitioner's name: *(in capitals/stamp)*
Date: / /	
Ophthalmic list number:	

Name or code of Health Authority receiving GOS 1 form for this sight test:

GOS 2

Part 3   Patient's information

The doctor or optometrist who tested your sight will tell you if this is a new or changed prescription, and if you need glasses. If so, you can have this prescription dispensed by an optician of your choice, but not all opticians can supply contact lenses. Unregistered suppliers may not sell glasses to anyone under 16 or anyone registered blind or partially sighted. Unregistered suppliers may not sell contact lenses.

About the NHS optical voucher

If you are in one of the groups below when you order your glasses or contact lenses, ask for an optical voucher when you have your sight test. Fill in Part 1 of the voucher form and give it to the optician.

If you were not entitled to a voucher when you had your sight test, but think you may be now, you can ask for one from the optician who is to supply your glasses. If they do not have vouchers, you can go back to the person who tested your sight and ask for a voucher before you order your glasses or contact lenses.

Your entitlement to help

You are entitled to the full value of a voucher *if, at the time you order* your glasses or contact lenses:

- you are under 16
- you are aged 16, 17 or 18 in full-time education
- you or your partner (if you have one) are getting:
    - Income Support
    - Income-based Jobseeker's Allowance
    - full Working Families' Tax Credit *or* Credit reduced by £70 or less
    - full Disabled Person's Tax Credit *or* Credit reduced by £70 or less
- you or your partner hold an HC2 certificate for full help

If you are not in one of the groups above, but you were prescribed complex lenses, you are also entitled to some help.

If you were given a voucher when you had your sight test but your circumstances change before you order your glasses/contact lenses, you cannot use your voucher unless you are still in one of the above groups when you order your glasses/contact lenses.

You may also be entitled to some help if you or your partner hold an HC3 certificate.

The value of your NHS optical voucher

The value of your voucher depends on your prescription and will match a letter from A to H, plus supplements (if any). Your optician has marked the letter and supplements on this form and the voucher form and can tell you the current values. Voucher values and supplements are also listed in leaflet HC12 *'NHS charges and optical voucher values'*. Ask your optician for a copy or get one from a Social Security office or main Post Office. You will be asked to provide evidence of your eligibility for a voucher.

GOS 3 NHS optical voucher and patient's statement

To get your glasses/contact lenses, fill in, sign and date Part 1 when you order them from the optician of your choice. Sign and date Part 2 overleaf to confirm that you have received them.

NHS optical voucher

* delete as appropriate

Mr/Mrs/Miss/Ms*:   Previous surname:

Other names: Date of birth: /   /

Address:

Postcode:

 # if known

Date of this prescription: /   /   NHS no#:   N.I.no#:

To be completed by the practitioner at your sight test

Voucher type: ☐   Supplements: ✓☐ *Complex* ✓☐ *Prism* ✓☐ *Tint*

R I G H T	Sph	Cyl	Axis	Prism	Base		Sph	Cyl	Axis	Prism	Base	L E F T
						Distance						
						Near						

† if applicable

Health Authority receiving relevant GOS1†:

Practitioner's name: *(print)*   Ophthalmic list no:

Signature: Date: /   /

Part 1 Patient's statement

My name and address are as shown above. I wish to order glasses/contact lenses* and I am entitled to use the above voucher today because:

Optician's use only
Evidence not seen

Tick any box which applies to you. These circumstances must apply on the date you order your glasses or contact lenses

✓☐ I am under 16

✓☐ I am a full time student aged 16, 17 or 18 and attend:

School/College/University*:

Address:

Postcode:

I/my* partner receive(s):

✓☐ Income Support   ✓☐ Income-based Jobseeker's Allowance

✓☐ Working Families' Tax Credit   ✓☐ Disabled Person's Tax Credit
(maximum rate *or* reduced by £70 or less)   (maximum rate *or* reduced by £70 or less)

Person getting the benefit/Credit* if not the patient:

Name: Date of birth: /   /

I/my* partner have ✓☐ HC2 ✓☐ HC3 certificate number:
The HC3 **(box B)** shows that the voucher value will be reduced by: £

✓☐ I have been prescribed complex lenses under the NHS optical voucher scheme

I declare that the information given on this form is correct and complete and I understand that if it is not, appropriate action may be taken. I confirm proper entitlement to an NHS optical voucher and for the purpose of checking this, I consent to the disclosure of relevant information, including to and by the Inland Revenue and Local Authorities.

** If you are under 16 or incapable of signing, your parent, carer or other person responsible for you should sign and give their name in capitals

I am the ✓☐ patient ✓☐ patient's carer or guardian.

Signature**:   Date: /   /

NOV. 00

NHS

GOS 3

Part 2 Supplier's declaration

In accordance with the prescription overleaf I have supplied:

[✓] glasses or   [✓] contact lenses because the patient named on this optical voucher:

[✓] requires a new or changed prescription

[✓] has an unchanged prescription but glasses/contact lenses* which are unserviceable due to fair wear and tear

* delete as appropriate

CLAIM

I claim under the NHS optical voucher scheme as follows:

	1st pair		2nd pair	
Actual cost of glasses/contact lenses* if less than or equal to voucher value(s) plus any supplement(s)	£	+	£	(1)
Voucher value(s)	£		£	(2)

Supplement(s)

1st pair		2nd pair				
[✓] Complex	[✓] Complex	£		£		(3)
[✓] Prism	[✓] Prism	£		£		(4)
[✓] Tint	[✓] Tint	£		£		(5)
[✓] Small glasses†	[✓] Small glasses†	£		£		(6)

†Please state boxed centre distance in millimetres

	1st pair		2nd pair	
Total of voucher(s) and supplement(s) *(sum of 2,3,4, 5+6)*	£	+	£	(7)
The cost of the glasses or contact lenses exceeds (7) for the	[✓] 1st pair		[✓] 2nd pair	
Maximum claimable for glasses/contact lenses* *(lower of 1 or 7)*	£			(8)
Patient's contribution as shown by **box B** of HC3 *(if applicable)*	£			(9)
Total claim for glasses/contact lenses* *(8 minus 9)*	£			

I declare that the information given on this form is correct and complete and I understand that if it is not, action may be taken against me. For the purpose of verification of this claim, I consent to the disclosure of relevant information. I claim payment of fees due to me for work carried out under the NHS optical voucher scheme.

Supplier's signature:

Supplier's name and address: *(in capitals/stamp)*

Date of first/only pair supplied: /   /

Date of second pair supplied: /   /

HA supplier code:

Part 3 Patient's declaration

I confirm that I have received [ ] pair(s) of glasses/contact lenses on [Date(s)   /   /   ] under the NHS optical voucher scheme. I declare that the information given on this form is correct and complete and I understand that if it is not, action may be taken against me.

I am the [✓] patient   [✓] patient's carer or guardian.

** If you are under 16 or incapable of signing, your parent, carer or other person responsible for you should sign

Signature**:   Date: /   /

Name: *(in block capitals)*

Address: *(if different from overleaf)*

Postcode:

Note

If you are a War Pensioner and need glasses because of your pensionable disability, send your prescription and receipt to: *War Pensions Agency, Norcross, Blackpool FY8 3WP*. Tell them your War Pension reference number.

GOS 4 NHS optical repair/replacement voucher application form

Fill in your details at Part 1, sign it and date Part 2 and give the form to the person who will repair or replace your glasses or contact lenses (more information is in leaflet HC11).

You cannot get help if your glasses/contact lenses are covered by warranty, insurance or after care service. If they were not, and you are aged 16 or over, you must satisfy the Health Authority that your glasses or contact lenses were lost or damaged because you were ill. You can wait for the Health Authority to approve your claim before you get the repair/replacement done or you can pay and claim a refund. But you can only have a refund if your Health Authority agrees.

Part 1 Patient's details

* delete as appropriate

Mr/Mrs/Miss/Ms*:   Previous surname:

Other names: Date of birth: /   /

Address:

                                                    Postcode:

 # if known Date of last NHS sight test: /   /   NHS no#:   N.I.no#:

Tick any box which applies to you to tell us the reason why you are entitled to a voucher

☑ I am under 16 (go to Part 2)

☑ I am a full time student aged 16, 17 or 18

I/my* partner receive(s):

☑ Income Support   ☑ Income-based Jobseeker's Allowance

☑ Working Families' Tax Credit   ☑ Disabled Person's Tax Credit
(maximum rate *or* reduced by £70 or less)   (maximum rate *or* reduced by £70 or less)

Person getting the benefit/Credit* if not the patient:

Name: Date of birth: /   /

I/my* partner have ☑ HC2   ☑ HC3 certificate number:

The HC3 (**box B**) shows that the voucher value will be reduced by: £

† Without this explanation the Health Authority cannot decide if you can have help

☑ I have been prescribed complex lenses as defined for the purposes of the NHS voucher scheme

☑ I have explained below† how the loss or damage happened.

Optician's use only
Evidence not seen

Part 2 Patient's declaration

I declare that the information given on this form is correct and complete and I understand that if it is not, appropriate action may be taken. I confirm proper entitlement to an NHS optical repair/replacement voucher and for the purpose of checking this, I consent to the disclosure of relevant information, including to and by the Inland Revenue and Local Authorities.

There is no insurance warranty or after sales service covering these glasses or contact lenses.

I agree to repay the voucher value if I am later found not to be entitled.

I am the ☑ patient   ☑ patient's carer or guardian.

** If you are under 16 or incapable of signing, your parent, carer or other person responsible for you should sign.

Signature**:   Date: /   /

Name: *(in block capitals)*

Address: *(if different from above)*

                                                    Postcode:

NOV. 00

NHS

GOS 4

Part 3   To be completed by the Health Authority

The applicant's claim has been considered and is:

[✓] approved   [✓] not approved

Health Authority name and address:
(stamp or write in capitals)

Signature: Date: /   /

Part 4   Patient's declaration

** *If you are under 16 or incapable of signing, your parent, carer or other person responsible for you should sign*

I confirm that my glasses/contact lenses* have been [✓] repaired [✓] replaced

I am the [✓] patient [✓] patient's carer or guardian

Signature**:   Date: /   /

Part 5   Supplier's declaration

* *delete as appropriate*

In accordance with the prescription and details below I have:

[✓] repaired [✓] replaced the glasses/contact lenses* for the person named at Part 1 of this form.

To be completed by the supplier where new lens(es) are required

RIGHT	Sph	Cyl	Axis	Prism	Base		Sph	Cyl	Axis	Prism	Base	LEFT
						Distance						
						Near						

Voucher type: [ ]   Supplements: [✓] *Complex* [✓] *Prism* [✓] *Tint*

Voucher value appropriate to the above prescription   £ _____ (1)

Parts: Lens/C.L* [✓] *Right* [✓] *Left* [✓] *Both*   £ _____ (2)

        Frame [✓] *Front* [✓] *Side* [✓] *Whole*   £ _____ (3)

Supplements: [✓] *Complex*   £ _____ (4)

             [✓] *Prism*   £ _____ (5)

             [✓] *Tint*   £ _____ (6)

             [✓] *Small glasses*   £ _____ (7)

CLAIM

I claim under the NHS optical voucher scheme:

Voucher value plus any supplement(s) *(sum of 1+(4+5+6+7))*   £ _____ (8)

or part(s) per current FPN plus any supplement(s) *(sum of (2+3)+(4+5+6+7))*   £ _____ (9)

or actual retail cost, if less   £ _____ (10)

Patient's contribution as shown by **box B** of certificate HC3 *(if applicable)*   £ _____ (11)

Total claim *(8 or 9 or 10 – whichever is the lowest, minus 11)*   £ _____

I declare that the information given on this form is correct and complete and I understand that if it is not, action may be taken against me. For the purpose of verification of this claim, I consent to the disclosure of relevant information. I claim payment of fees due to me for work carried out under the NHS optical voucher scheme.

Supplier's signature: Supplier's name and address:
(in capitals/stamp)

Date: /   /

HA supplier code:

GOS 5 Help with the cost of a private sight test

If you (or your partner) hold an HC3 certificate for limited help with health costs, you may be able to get help with the cost of a private sight test. More information is in leaflet HC11. If you think you might be entitled to help with the cost of your glasses, ask when you have your sight test.

Part 1 Patient's details

* delete as appropriate

Mr/Mrs/Miss/Ms*:   P   revious surname:

Other names: Date of birth: /   /

Address:

Postcode:

 # if known   Date of last NHS sight test: /   /   NHS no#:   N.I.no#:

Reason for patient's entitlement to vouchers

✓   I/my* partner have HC3 certificate number:

–showing (at **box A**) that I have to pay up to   £   for a private sight test.

I will pay up to the amount above (plus any difference between the NHS sight test fee and the cost of my private sight test) provided my private sight test cost more than the NHS sight test.

Note: The person who tests your sight can tell you the NHS sight test fee. This is also in leaflet HC12 *'NHS charges and optical voucher values'*. Ask your optician for a copy or get one from a Social Security office or main Post Office.

✓   I have had a sight test at home because I cannot leave home unaccompanied

Part 2 Patient's declaration

This is my application for help with the cost of a private sight test.

I declare that the information given on this form is correct and complete and I understand that if it is not, appropriate action may be taken. I confirm proper entitlement to help with the cost of a private sight test and for the purpose of checking this, I consent to the disclosure of relevant information, including to and by the Inland Revenue and Local Authorities.

I am the   ✓   patient   ✓   patient's carer or guardian.

**If you are incapable of signing, your parent, carer or other person responsible for you should sign and give their name

Signature**:   Date: /   /

Name: *(in block capitals)*

Address: *(if different from above)*

Postcode:

NOV. 00

NHS

GOS 5

Part 3   **Practitioner's declaration**

I declare that I have tested the sight of the patient overleaf on *(date)*   /   /

✓ The patient was referred to their GP
✓ A prescription showing no change *or* a statement was issued
✓ A new or changed prescription was issued
✓ A voucher was issued:

Voucher type: [ ]   Supplements: ✓ *Complex*   ✓ *Prism*   ✓ *Tint*

This patient was the:

✓ 1st patient at that address
✓ 2nd patient at that address
✓ 3rd or subsequent patient at that address

This patient was unable to attend the practice for their sight test because:

CLAIM   I claim for a sight test:

Lower of private charge or NHS sight test fee __	£	(1)
Lower of the private charge or NHS domiciliary visit fee *(where appropriate)*	£	(2)
Maximum claimable in respect of sight test *(sum of 1+2)*	£	(3)
Patient's contribution as shown by **box A** of HC3	£	(4)
Total claim in respect of sight test *(3 minus 4)*	£	

Address where sight test took place: *(in capitals/stamp)*

Address *(if different)* where payment should be sent: *(in capitals/stamp)*

I declare that the information given on this form is correct and complete and I understand that if it is not, action may be taken against me. For the purpose of verification of this claim, I consent to the disclosure of relevant information. I claim payment of fees due to me for work carried out under the NHS optical voucher scheme.

Practitioner's signature:

Practitioner's name: *(in capitals/stamp)*

Date: /   /

Ophthalmic list number:

Optical Bodies and Associations

American Academy of Optometry (British Chapter)

This is an affiliated chapter of the American Academy based in the UK open to UK optometrists who meet the requirements of the American Academy.

> Andrew Field
> 2 Doric Lodge
> Doric Place
> Woodbridge
> Suffolk IP12 1BT
> www.academy.org.uk

Association of British Dispensing Opticians (ABDO)

The ABDO represents qualified dispensing opticians. A regular magazine *Dispensing Optics* is published.

> 6 Hurlingham Business Park
> Sulivan Road
> London SW6 3DU
> Tel.: 020 8736 0088

Association of Contact Lens Manufacturers

Representing the major manufacturers of contact lenses in the UK.

> Simon Rodwell
> PO Box 737
> Devizes
> Wilts SN10 3TQ
> www.aclm.org.uk

Association of Optometrists (AOP)

The AOP represents the political interests of the optometrist. Approximately half of all qualified optometrists are members. A regular magazine *Optometry Today* is published.

> 61 Southwark Street
> London SE1 0HL
> Tel.: 020 7261 9661
> www.assoc-optometrists.org

British Contact Lens Association

Ophthalmic opticians/optometrists and dispensing opticians with a special interest in contact lenses may join this association. A regular journal is published.

> Walmar House
> 288–292 Regent Street
> London W1R 5HF

Tel.: 020 7580 6669
www.bcla.org.uk

Department of Health
Richmond House
79 Whitehall
SW1A 2NS
Tel.: 020 7210 3000

Eye Care Trust
PO Box 131
Market Rasen
Lincolnshire LN8 5TS

College of Optometrists (COptom)
Representing over 90% of qualified optometrists, the college maintains
professional standards, organizes professional examinations and monitors
the academic standards of the profession. A journal, *Ophthalmic* and *Physiological Optics*, is published four times a year.
42 Craven Street
London WC2 5NG
Tel.: 020 7839 6000
www.college-optometrists.org

Federation of Ophthalmic and Dispensing Opticians
This organization represents registered opticians in business.
113 Eastbourne Mews
London W2 6LQ
Tel.: 020 7258 0240
www.fodo.com

General Optical Council (GOC)
Established under the terms of the Opticians Act 1958, the GOC has a duty
to protect the public interest by setting required standards for the
ophthalmic optical/optometric profession.
41 Harley Street
London W1N 2DJ
Tel.: 020 7580 3898
www.optical.org

Institute of Optometry
A registered charity providing eye care services, clinical research and post-
graduate training.
56–62 Newington Causeway
London SE1 6DS
Tel.: 020 7407 4183
www.ioo.org.uk

Royal College of Ophthalmologists
Representing consultants in ophthalmology and those studying for specialist
qualifications in ophthalmology.
17 Cornwall Terrace
London NW1 4QW
Tel.: 020 7935 0702

Scottish Committee of Optometrists (SCO)
Arranges meetings, lectures and remains active politically in Scottish optical affairs.

7 Queens Buildings
Queensferry Road
Rosyth KY11 2RA
Tel.: 01383 419444

Worshipful Company of Spectacle Makers (SMC)
The oldest established of the remaining professional organizations, this company now has forsaken its examining role in optometry, and has become more involved with training in the optical manufacturing industry.

Apothecaries Hall
Blackfriars Lane
London EC4V 6EL
Tel.: 020 7236 2932

References and Further Reading

Statutes

Partnership Act 1890
Sale of Goods Act 1893
Limited Partnerships Act 1907
Registration of Business Names Act 1916
Factories Act 1937
National Health Service Act 1946
National Health Service (Scotland) Act 1947
Health Services (Northern Ireland) Act 1947
Nurseries and Child-Minders Regulation Act 1948
National Assistance Act 1948
Companies Act 1948
National Health Service (Amendment) Act 1949
Shops Act 1950
National Health Service Act 1951
National Health Service Act 1952
Opticians Act 1958
Factories Act 1961
National Health Service Act 1961
Offices, Shops and Railway Premises Act 1963
Shops (Early Closing Days) Act 1965
Companies Act 1967
Misrepresentation Act 1967
Trade Descriptions Act 1968
Health Services and Public Health Act 1968
Medicines Act 1968
Employers Liability (Compulsory Insurance) Act 1969
Equal Pay Act 1970
Misuse of Drugs Act 1971
Fire Precautions Act 1971
Road Traffic Act 1972

National Health Service Reorganisation Act 1973
Health and Safety at Work etc. Act 1974
Sex Discrimination Act 1975
National Health Service Act 1977
Criminal Law Act 1977
National Health Service (Scotland) Act 1978
Employment Protection (Consolidation) Act 1978
Sale of Goods Act 1979
Health Service Act 1980
Supreme Court Act 1981
Supply of Goods and Services Act 1982
Health and Social Security Act 1984
Data Protection Act 1984
Companies Consolidation (Consequential Provisions) Act 1985
National Health Service (Amendment) Act 1986
Health and Medicines Act 1988
Opticians Act 1989
National Health Service and Community Care Act 1990
Access to Health Records Act 1990
Sale and Supply of Goods Act 1994
Health Authorities Act 1995
Disability Discrimination Act 1995
Employment Rights Act 1996
The National Health Service (Primary Care) Act 1997
Data Protection Act 1998
Health Act 1999

Statutory instruments

1922/731   Chemical Works Regulations
1953/1464 Iron and Steel Foundries Regulations
1956/1077 National Health Service (Service Committees and Tribunal) Regulations
1956/1078 National Health Service (Supplementary Ophthalmic Services) Regulations
1960/1932 Shipbuilding and Ship-Repairing Regulations
1960/1934 General Optical Council (Disciplinary Committee Roles) Order of Council
1960/1935 General Optical Council (Investigating Committee Rules) Order of Council
1960/1936 General Optical Council (Rules Relating to Injury or Disease of the Eye) Order of Council
1961/1239 General Optical Council Disciplinary Committee (Legal Assessor) Rules
1961/1580 Construction (General Provisions) Regulations
1961/1933 General Optical Council (Disciplinary Committee) Procedure Order of Council
1962/1667 Non-Ferrous Metals (Melting and Founding Regulations)
1964/167   General Optical Council (Rules on Publicity) Order of Council

1965/1366	National Health Service (Service Committees and Tribunal) Amendment Regulations
1969/354	National Health Service (Service Committees and Tribunal) (Amendment) Regulations
1969/1826	General Optical Council (Disciplinary Committee) (Procedure) Order of Council
1974/287	National Health Service (General Ophthalmic Services) Regulations
1974/455	National Health Service (Service Committees and Tribunal) Regulations
1974/527	National Health Service (General Ophthalmic Services) (Amendment) Regulations
1974/907	National Health Service (Service Committees and Tribunal) Amendment Regulations
1974/1681	Protection of Eyes Regulations
1975/789	(Section 129) National Health Service (General Ophthalmic Services) (S.) (Amendment) Regulations
1976/303	Protection of Eyes (Amendment) Regulations
1976/968	The Medicines (Specified Articles and Substances) Order
1976/2010	Fire Precautions (Non-certificated Factory, Office, Shop and Railway Premises) Regulations
1977/434	National Health Service (Charges and Remission) Amendment Regulations
1977/1999	National Health Service (General Ophthalmic Services) Amendment Regulations
1977/2127	Medicines (Prescription Only) Order
1977/2129	Medicines (General Sale List) Order
1977/2132	Medicines (Sale or Supply) (Miscellaneous Provisions) Regulations
1977/2133	Medicines (Pharmacy and General Sale – Exemption) Order
1978/950	National Health Service (Dental and Optical Charges) Regulations
1978/987	Medicines (Prescription Only) Amendment (No. 2) Order
1978/988	Medicines (Pharmacy and General Sale – Exemption) Amendment Order
1978/989	Medicines (Sale or Supply) (Miscellaneous Provisions) Amendment Regulations
1979/1114	Medicines (Exemption from Licences) (Assembly) Order
1979/1539	Medicines (Contact Lens Fluids and Other Substances) (Appointed Day) Order
1979/1585	Medicines (Contact Lens Fluids and Other Substances) (Exemption from Licences) Order
1980/1921	Medicines (Prescription Only) Order
1980/1922	Medicines (General Sale List) Order
1980/1923	Medicines (Sale or Supply) Miscellaneous Provisions Regulations
1980/1924	Medicines (Pharmacy and General Sale – Exemption) Order
1981/552	General Optical Council (Rules and Publicity) Order
1981/952	Motor Vehicle (Driving Licences) Regulations
1982/28	Medicines (Sale or Supply) (Miscellaneous Provisions) Amendment Regulations

1983/1212	Medicines (Products other than Veterinary Drugs) (Prescription Only) Order
1984/769	Medicines (Products other than Veterinary Drugs) (General Sales List) Order
1984/1778	Sale of Optical Appliances Order
1985/203	General Optical Council (Rules on Publicity) Order
1985/1298	National Health Service (General Ophthalmic Services) Amendment Regulations
1985/856	General Optical Council (Rules on Fitting Contact Lenses) Order
1985/2024	General Optical Council (Registration and Enrolment) (Amendment) (Rules) Order
1986/309	General Optical Council (Membership) Order
1986/974	Health and Social Security Act 1984 (Commencement No. 2) Order
1986/975	National Health Service (General Ophthalmic Service) Regulations
1986/976	National Health Service (Payments for Optical Appliances) Regulations
1986/1136	National Health Service (Payments for Optical Appliances) Amendment Regulations
1988/428	National Health Service (Payments for Optical Appliances) Regulations
1988/486	National Health Service (General Ophthalmic Services) Amendment Regulations
1988/552	National Health Service (Payments for Optical Appliances) Amendment No. 2 Regulations
1988/1305	General Optical Council (Contact Lens (Qualifications, etc.) (Rules)) Order
1989/375	General Optical Council (Contact Lens (Qualifications, etc.) ((Amendment) Rules)) Order of Council
1989/395	National Health Service (General Ophthalmic Services) Amendment Regulations
1989/1230	Sight Testing (Examination and Prescription) (No. 2) Regulations
1989/1174	The Health and Medicines Act 1988 (Commencement No. 5) Order
1989/1175	National Health Service (General Ophthalmic Services) Amendment No. 2 Regulations
1989/1176	Sight Testing (Examination and Prescription) Regulations General Optical Council (Specification) Rules Order of Council
1989/1852	Medicines (Prescription Only, Pharmacy and General Sale) Amendment Order
1990/495	National Health Service (Optical Charges and Payments) Amendment Regulations
1990/538	National Health Service (Service Committees and Tribunal) Amendment Regulations
1990/1051	The National Health Service (General Ophthalmic Services) Amendment Regulations
1990/1752	National Health Service, (Service Committees and Tribunal) Amendment (No. 2) Regulations
1991/824	European Communities (Recognition of Professional Qualifications) Regulations

1992/664	National Health Service (Service Committees and Tribunal) Regulations
1993/483	General Optical Council (Registration and Enrolment (Amendment) Rules)
1994/70	General Optical Council (Testing of Sight by Persons Training as Ophthalmic Opticians Rules)
1994/2579	General Optical Council (Companies Committee Rules) Order of Council
1995/558	National Health Service (General Ophthalmic Services) Amendment Regulations
1995/3091	National Health Service (Service Committees and Tribunal) Amendment Regulations
1996/703	National Health Service (Service Committees and Tribunal) Amendment Regulations
1996/705	National Health Service (General Ophthalmic Services) Amendment Regulations
1996/2320	National Health Service (General Ophthalmic Services) Amendment (No.) Regulations
1996/2374	European Communities (Recognition of Professional Qualifications) (Second General System) Regulations
1997/818	National Health Service (Optical Charges and Payments) Regulations
1997/1780	National Health Service (Primary Care) Act 1997 (Commencement No. 1) Order
1997/1830	Prescription only Medicines (Human Use) Order
1998/1338	General Optical Council (Disciplinary Committee (Constitution) Rules)
1998/1337	General Optical Council (Disciplinary Committee (Procedure) (Amendment) Rules)
1998/3117	General Optical Council (Membership)
1999/609	National Health Service (Optical Charges and Payments) Amendment Regulations
1999/693	National Health Service (General Ophthalmic Services) (Amendment) Regulations
1999/1211	General Optical Council (Education Committee Rules)
1999/2562	National Health Service (Optical Charges and Payments) and (General Ophthalmic Services) (Amendment) Regulations
1999/2801	Commission for Health Improvement (Membership and Procedure) Regulations
1999/2897	General Optical Council (Testing of Sight by Persons Training as Ophthalmic Opticians Rules) (Amendment)
1999/3267	General Optical Council (Rules relating to Injury or Disease of the Eye)
2000/89	Primary Care Trusts (Membership, Procedure and Administration Arrangements) Regulations

Books and journals

Angel S and Taylor SP (1999) Professional insurance cover. *Optician* 218(5690), 20–22

Carey P (1998) *Data Protection Act*. Blackstone Press, London

Classe JG (1989) *Legal Aspects of Optometry*. Butterworths, Boston, USA

Cole J (1979) The Thiriart Report – an assessment of optometry in Europe. *Optician* 17, May 11, 13–17

Drasdo N and Haggerty CM (1981) A comparison of the British number-plate and Snellen vision test for car drivers. *Ophthalmic and Physiological Optics* 1, 39–54

Doughty MJ (1999) *Drugs, Medications and the Eye*. Butterworth-Heinemann

Giles GH (1953) The Ophthalmic Services under the National Health Service Acts 1946–1952. Hammonds, London

Grit F (2000) Optometry in the Netherlands. *Optometry Today* 41, 3

Hofstetter HW (1976) Optometry on the Continent, 2, Belgium. *Optician* 172, October 8, 8–9

Hofstetter HW (1976) Optometry on the Continent, 3, Denmark. *Optician* 172, October 22, 25–27

Hofstetter HW (1976) Optometry on the Continent, 6, France. *Optician* 172, December 10, 13–15

Hofstetter HW (1976) Optometry on the Continent, 7, Italy. *Optician* 172, December 24–31, 16–25

Hofstetter HW (1977) Optometry on the Continent, 8, Netherlands. *Optician* 173, January 28, 11–15

Hofstetter HW (1977) Optometry on the Continent, 11, West Germany. *Optician* 173, March 25, 18–35

Hopkins G and Pearson R (1998) *Ophthalmic Drugs*. Butterworth-Heinemann

Koch CC (1947) British reaction to the national health insurance scheme. *American Journal of Optometrists and Archives of the Academy of Optometrists* 24, 151–169

North RV (1999) *Work and the Eye*. Butterworth-Heinemann

O'Connor Davies PH (1978) Medicines legislation and the ophthalmic optician. *Ophthalmic Optician* 18, 688–694

O'Connor Davies PH (1980) The use of ophthalmic drugs in the UK. *American Journal of Optometry and Physiological Optics* 57, 925–926

Office of Fair Trading (1982) *Opticians and Competition*. HMSO, London

Redmond PWD (1970) *General Principles of English Law*. Macdonald & Evans, London

Roussell DF (1979) *Eye Protection*. Royal Society for the Prevention of Accidents, Birmingham

Seaton CN (1966) *Aspects of the National Health Service Acts*. Pergamon Press, Oxford

Simmonds AB (1981) The attitude of the public towards the optometric profession. *Optician* 181, June 26, 22–28

Solomons H (1991) Computers: taking stock. *The Optician* February 8, 20–30

Taylor SP (1982) Ophthalmic law. *Optician* 188(4757), 10

Taylor SP (1983) New York State optometry: its legislation and practice. *Optician* 186(4820), 11–12

Taylor SP (1984) Advertising – a professional spectacle. *Optician* 187(4930), 10–13

Taylor SP (1986) The effect of the Health and Social Security Act 1988, on the profession of optometry in the UK. *American Journal of Optometry and Physiological Optics* 63, 377–381

Taylor SP (1991) The Opticians Act 1989 and UK Optometry. *Ophthalmic and Physiological Optics* 11, 185–190

Taylor SP (1991) The OSAC and UK Optometry. *Ophthalmic and Physiological Optics* 11, 271–274

Taylor SP (1994) The Health and Safety (Display Screen Equipment) Regulations 1992. *Ophthalmic and Physiological Optics* 14, 210–212

Taylor SP (1998) The negligent professional. *Optician* 216(5682), 26–27

Taylor SP and Edwards KH (1998) Fitness to practise procedure. *Optician* 217(5685), 32–34

Walding N and Laundy P (1961) *An Encyclopaedia of Parliament*. Cassell, London

Yarmocsky R (1984) The legal diversification of optometry. *Journal of the American Optometric Association* 55, 665–669

Yeomans F (1984) Optometry in West Germany. *Optician* 188(4966), 31–35

Reports

Report of the Committee appointed by the Minister of Health and the Secretary of State for Scotland on the Optical Practitioners (Registration) Bill 1927: December 1927; Cmnd 2999, HMSO, London

Report of the Eye Services Committee to the Ophthalmic Sub-committee of the Negotiating Committee of the Medical Profession and the Joint Emergency Committee of the Optical Profession: May 1947, Ministry of Health

Report of the Interdepartmental Committee on the Statutory Registration of Opticians: April 1952; Cmnd 8531, HMSO, London

Price Commission report on prices of private spectacles and contact lenses: August 1976; Report No. 20, HMSO, London

Opticians and Competition: December 1982; HMSO, London

Primary Health Care, an agenda for discussion: April 1986; Cmnd 9771, HMSO, London

The Government's Competition Policies and Optometry: 1987; London, Association of Optometrists

The Future of the Profession of Optometry: 1989: London, British College of Optometrists

Report of the review of optical services undertaken by the Optical Services Audit Committee: 1990; London, General Optical Council

Vision for Optics in 2000. April 1990; Henley Centre

Review of Prescribing, Supply and Administration of Medicines Part 1 1998

Review of Prescribing, Supply and Administration of Medicines Final Report 1999

Professional/government publications

AOP. Starting an Optometric Practice 1999

AOP. The Eye Examination and Related Matters 1999

AOP, ABDO & FODO. Making Accurate Claims 1999

College of Optometrists. Optometrists' Formulary Number 3 1998

College of Optometrists. Primary Eye Care Services 1999

College of Optometrists. Clinical Audit Framework for Optometric Practice 2001

College of Optometrists. Code of Ethics and Guidelines for Professional Conduct 2001

Department of Health. The New NHS 1997

Department of Health. A First Class Service 1998

Department of Health. The NHS Plan 2000

FODO. Optics at a Glance 1985–2000

NHS. Executive Complaints – Guidance Pack for Optometrists 1996

NHS. Executive Primary Care: The Future 1996

NHS. Executive Action on Cataracts 2000

NHS. Executive Optical Point of Service Checks in England 2001

Index